YOGA LESSONS FOR DEVELOPING SPIRITUAL CONSCIOUSNESS

BY

SWAMIE A. P. MUKERJI

First published in 1911

Published by Left of Brain Books

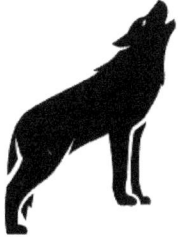

Copyright © 2023 Left of Brain Books

ISBN 978-1-396-32328-7

First Edition

All rights reserved. No part of this publication may be reproduced, distributed, or transmitted in any form or by any means, including photocopying, recording, or other electronic or mechanical methods, without the prior written permission of the publisher, except in the case of brief quotations permitted by copyright law. Left of Brain Books is a division of Left Of Brain Onboarding Pty Ltd.

PUBLISHER'S PREFACE

About the Book

"This is one of the Yogi Publication Society (YPS) titles, which may have been in part or whole written by William Walker Atkinson. At the very least, this volume seems to have been padded out a bit. The first few chapters are consistent in tone and style, and discuss basics of Hindu (or perhaps Theosophist) thought in very general terms, with lots of italics and small caps for emphasis. There is even a realistic description of a saddhu and a fishmarket in Benares, local color which you don't typically find in the YPS series. Hindu technical terms are used correctly (and spelled correctly)."

(Quote from sacred-texts.com)

CONTENTS

PUBLISHER'S PREFACE
INTRODUCTION 1
   THE YOGI CONCEPTION OF LIFE 2
   THE IDEAL AND THE PRACTICAL 6
   READ AND REFLECT 9
   MAN: ANIMAL AND DIVINE 12
   DOUBLE CONSCIOUSNESS 16
   SPIRITUAL UNFOLDMENT 19
   CAUSE AND EFFECT 24
   MAN—THE MASTER 29
   SELF-DEVELOPMENT 33
   DEVELOPING THE SPIRITUAL CONSCIOUSNESS 36
   WHO CAN BE A YOGI? 45
   CONSTRUCTIVE IDEALISM 53
   HIGHER REASON AND JUDGMENT 60
   CONQUEST OF FEAR 66
   THE ROLE OF PRAYER 69
   THOUGHT: CREATIVE AND EXHAUSTIVE 77
   MEDITATION EXERCISE 85
   SELF-DE-HYPNOTISATION 91
   SELF-DE-HYPNOTISATION—II 94
   CHARACTER-BUILDING 106
   CONCLUSION 115

INTRODUCTION

VERILY, in whom unwisdom is destroyed by the wisdom of the Self, in them, Wisdom, shining as the Sun, reveals the Supreme.—BHAGAVAD GITA.

Yoga is a subject which has enthralled the attention of the world from time out of mind. No one has hitherto done justice to such a grand system though there have been, now and then, innumerable attempts.

The present author, my esteemed friend, Swami Mukerji, a Yogi who comes out of a successive generation of Yogis, is a fit and proper instrument to handle the subject. He, in these lessons prepares the layman for an understanding of the Yoga and, through a series of wise and masterful sayings, impresses on the mind of the reader the necessity for rising above materialism, nay, solves the very problem "What am I?"

Every line is pregnant with mature thoughts and rivets one's attention, and makes him think, think, think.

This is not a work for which an introduction, briefly setting forth the contents, could be written.

I can but ask you to read, digest and improve.

DR. T. R. SANJIVI, PH.D.,
President,
THE LATENT LIGHT CULTURE.

Tinnevelly, India.

THE YOGI CONCEPTION OF LIFE

IF we study the action of mind upon mind, of mind over matter, of mind over the human body, we may realize how "each man is a power in himself"—to use Mr. Randall's phrase in his beautiful book on psychology.

Life is demonstrative: it speaks with a million, million tongues. Life stands for Light and Love. Contemplation of Death, which is really a change, will not lead to Happiness.

All-stagnation is death. Humanity is a moving mass, and this is true of it as regards single units as well as of the collective whole.

Stop we cannot. We must go forwards, which is "God-wards" or there is the backward line of progress—which is IGNORANCE.

Spasms of activity catch hold of us and push us onward and, similarly, fear, weakness and worry, the triple weapons of our Old Friend, the Devil, catch us in their deadly grip and "crib, cabin and confine" us.

We all are preparing to live, day in and day out. Is it not so? The body ages; the soul is ever on the alert. We all are trying to grasp life in its proper perspective, to get a clear view of the goal ahead.

Some say "I am for enjoying life;" some say, "It is a bad mixture of heaven and hell, for the most part, hell;" others stand on neutral ground and say, "Let us make the best of a bad bargain. Since we are here, it is no use grumbling. This world is for our education."

Right. Move we must. It may be progress forward or progress backwards.

Life is a series of awakenings. Ideas dawn upon the mind from time to time, are caught up by brain and body and find physical expression as acts. Our outward life with its environment is fitted to our inward development. Wealth, position, fame, power,—all these are the simple expressions of individual character. This is not a platitude. Look and see for yourself.

It is quite necessary that we should pass through certain experiences, that we rise from ideal to ideal. We create our own fate. Our sufferings, our joys, are so many projections from ourselves. We alone are responsible for them.

Like the silkworm we build a cocoon around the soul and then feeling "Cramped," we set to loosening the bonds.

Enjoyment is not, ought not to be the goal of life. Sense-enjoyments end in satiety and exhaustion. Power and self, riches and all that riches mean, may tie us down to a narrow sphere. But in the long run we do come to know that happiness is not in them. This is a tremendous truth, yet God mercifully screens it from us till we are prepared to receive it.

What remains then? Man wants happiness. He rushes from one thing to another to grasp it, only to find everything slipping through his fingers. Let none deny it. "The aim of philosophy is to put an end to pain." All pain is caused by IGNORANCE. Apply the saving remedy of KNOWLEDGE, and PAIN vanishes at once. This is a great fact and all young men ought to stamp it well upon their minds.

While we are upon this phase of our subject, it may be worth while to go farther into these important facts of life—PLEASURE and PAIN.

Our thoughts and actions are the forces we send out of ourselves. All life is expression. The soul of man is trying to see itself in everything. How did the different organs of the body come into existence? How did man get his eyes, his ears, his nose and so forth? How does the growth of things proceed on the subconscious plane of existence? The soul willed to see and it saw, willed to hear and it heard, willed to smell and it smelt. That is the right explanation.

Take a subject, throw him into a hypnotic trance, lead him into the deepest state possible, give him vigorous suggestions that a steady increase is taking place as to his physique, repeat the suggestions twice every day for a few months and you will have put pounds of flesh on his form. If you know anything of these things at all, you will be hardly astonished. A striking case once occurred: Some frivolous students of Aberdeen held a hypnotic seance. A friend of theirs was hypnotised and made to go through certain illusions. Then a wet towel was put upon his neck and it was suggested to him that a sharp knife had been drawn right across his neck to cut his throat and that he was dead. It was such fun! The students danced for joy. But what was their surprise when they found the man was stone dead. It taught the eternal truth—what man thinks that he is, that he shall be.

Now, man is trying to express himself on the different planes of his being by appropriating to himself different vehicles of expression. When he meets with opposition, an obstacle, he chafes like a caged lion. Load the limbs of a man with fetters of iron and see the result. It is really this—when we can push forward without opposition, it causes pleasure, a sense of happiness; when we are held back it causes pain. Place good food before a healthy man. See how he likes it. It is because he knows that he is making an addition to himself. It brings on a sense of "MORE-NESS" and pleasure follows. Of course there are higher grades of this sense of "MORE-NESS." Some ancient doctors defined passion as an accession of strength due to the surcharge of arterial blood in the veins. All pleasure is from STRENGTH, all pain from WEAKNESS. There can be no question as to this fact.

There is a fire burning. Heap coals. The more coals, the brighter and steadier the flame. All obstacles are really "coal" feeding the "flame" of the spirit. They spur a man on. The vibrations of pain are often blessings in disguise. They drive the lesson home. The effect is not different from the cause. Both are the obverse and reverse of the same coin. Painful results grow out of deeds that clash with the interests of the DIVINITY WITHIN— which is for FREEDOM.

"Lord, I want nothing—neither health, nor beauty nor power. Give me FREEDOM and I am content." This is *Jivan mukti*. This is the highest ideal of life. Thinking of the little pleasures of the senses has brought us to this: to dance, to laugh, to weep, and before the tears are gone, to begin over again. Look at my condition. Slave of the flesh, slave of the mind, wanting to have this, that and what not. DARKNESS BEHIND—DARKNESS AHEAD. Such is the wail of IGNORANCE.

Get rid of it, O! My Friend. It is your greatest, direst enemy. Let the LIGHT of KNOWLEDGE dissipate this DARKNESS of IGNORANCE. The Lord above is our refuge. He alone is STRENGTH. "In Him we live and have our being." Where seek you for your ideals. Here it is. FREEDOM—You are rushing to it, and so am I. Welcome everything that helps you, yea, compels you, to strike one more blow in the noble cause of EMANCIPATION. "Can a marble figure brook the blow that an iron mass can bear." "Know, slave is slave, caressed or whipped. . . . Fetters, though of gold are not less strong to bind."

Thus, let us work it out. Let us cut short this show of five minutes with death and decay as its sequel. We shall go beyond this to the ONE SOURCE, GOD; and there is PEACE.

THE IDEAL AND THE PRACTICAL

HERE are two words—IMAGINATION and FANCY. What is the distinction between the two? Well, the one is closely related to the positive and the conscious side of our character; the other can claim kinship with the negative and the receptive side only. Take a youth starting in life. He has not been born with a silver spoon in his mouth. He is poor and has absolutely none to look to for help of any sort whatsoever.

Now, suppose *he has spirit*, and instead of sitting down and bewailing his lot, he forms a definite plan of conduct, throws his mind forward into the future, and decides to reach a certain state of development. He pictures to himself that state in its perfection, plans out the methods whereby he is to achieve it, takes in the difficulties to be met with and conquered, and by an effort of common sense reasoning sees the actual amount of good accruing to humanity and to all of God's creatures in general. He has had to think hard in order to construct the whole picture. He has had to breathe life upon it by repeating the images in connection with the whole picture. He has had to acquire knowledge, seek the advice of men more experienced than himself, and all the while he has had to keep up a brave and hopeful attitude of mind. And, mark you, he scorns to think of failure. It is for him to try his level best. It is for nature, which is a hard though a just pay-mistress, to bring him his reward in its due season.

The above is a fair example of the exercise of *Imagination*.

Fancy plays us tricks. It is not the man who pulls the strings this time. He simply yields himself to the influence of all sorts of impossible day-dreams. His mind is a sieve for thoughts to pass in and out. It is an aimless, idle, wandering, and brings ready victims for the "pitch-and-toss" game of men whose principle is to "*do*" others before the latter can have a turn at them.

A man is what his ideals are. If one man with an ideal makes fifty mistakes in a day, the man without an ideal is sure to commit many more. This is a simple truth, yet it will bear repetition here. All muscular actions, whether mental or physical, are simply fragments from the ideal.

"The life of the ideal is in the practical; it is the ideal that has penetrated the whole of our life, whether we philosophise or perform the hard, everyday duties of life. . . . It is the ideal that has made us what we are and will make us what we are to be. . . . The principle is seldom expressed in the practical, yet the ideal is never lost sight of"—("Pavhari Baba" by Vivekananda).

The very fact of the ideal being present in your mind foreshadows its fulfilment.

Our thoughts set up a magnetic centre within us. Like attracts like. Good thoughts draw to themselves corresponding thoughts. This fact is very emphatic. Each tree brings forth fruits of its kind. If we think *well*, we cannot act *ill*. The greatness of a man must find its measure in the greatness of his thoughts, and not in the amount of money in his pocket or the bluster on his tongue.

Our ideal is the hinge upon which our future turns. We create our own fate.

The first essential is to pitch our aims high. Let us look upward and upward alone. Let us pray to God for strength by all means, but let us be prepared to deserve His grace by walking a straight path.

If we weave our thoughts around a grand purpose in life the ideal so formed may take material form any day. Its impulsion may stir up concretions of gross physical matter into activity and may clap spurs to the feet of even a lazy hack. So much for the ideal.

If the ideal is to be *cherished*, it must also be *nourished*. If you simply sit down and desire to get a thing, you will never get it and it is good for you that you should not. For the practical side of things must never be neglected. "Practice makes perfect." Having set currents of holy desire in motion, we must set to deepen them in intensity and volume.

"Great actions are only transformed great concentrations."

Desire expands the will; action clinches it into strength. Each act in the right direction goes to establish us in our ideal. Action gives us training. Education is for self-discipline. Force of character is what we want; money, fame, praise and blame may well take care of themselves.

What matters it what the world thinks of me so long as I can think well of myself? Have I a clear conscience? Is my body under my control? Is my mind pure? Do I love main? Do I dare to look others straight in the eye? Do I fear anything?

The answer to such questions will go to make up the sum of our happiness or misery.

A strong will; a steady pulse; a pure mind; these are what we want.

But nought comes from nought—*Ex nihilo nihil fit*. Nothing will drop from the skies. See here, my brother, do you want a thing? Is it a good thing? *Then take it*. Let us deserve what we desire. That is the energetic way of setting about things.

Action, right action, unselfish action; these alone can give us strength. *To think is to act. To act is to live. To live is to love*. "Love, Love; that is the sole resource."

Therefore, O Thou Soul!, pray to thy primal source, God, for the power to make others happy.

Disease may come; limb after limb may be lopped off; sorrow may strike thee to the core; yet cease not to desire nobly, and to bear thyself in action yet more nobly.

The privacy of your own room, aye, of your own mind is the place where you must play the man.

We have long lived under the influence of fear—the firstborn of Ignorance. Let knowledge come and with it its power—Courage.

This is the supreme lesson we have to learn—Fear leads us from death to death; courage opens the gate into Life, Serenity, and Joy.

READ AND REFLECT

"WHATEVER is worth doing is worth doing well;"—an age-worn saying but one which cannot be rung too often on human ears. We are mostly selfish—and all blame to us!—and this because the Light of the Lord within us is so bedimmed by the darkness of the lower nature.

Our deeds are accomplished best when we put heart in them; when we see some gain accruing to us. Need I prove this?

What is the Central pivot we turn upon? Attraction;—and its opposite, Repulsion. We take an interest in certain things. The former gives us a touch of pleasure, the latter causes pain. Both act diametrically; and the will, unable to assert itself, is unable to draw to itself the happiness-giving objects. Pain racks the soul.

The aim of philosophy is to put an end to pain. It does not bring down upon us the gloom of despair, but the sunshine of Cheerfulness. Applying this to our actions we see how philosophy, in the *positive* sense, is a true helper. It hands us a *weapon* which cuts through difficulties. The weapon is *Wisdom*.

By Wisdom I mean a light which is *self-luminous*. Man has an *infinite* field of Consciousness. This sphere, as it widens out, realises for us all that we want *rightly*. Our actions become linked together symmetrically and at the end of the chain of wise activity is the *desired* object.

It is hence wise to acquire wisdom. How to do it? *By unfolding the consciousness*. How to unfold? Well, there are many methods, most difficult; but I am going to give you a very easy one, applying which, success is as sure as that morning follows night.

In the ordinary course of things we walk at a snail's pace, and progress is woefully slow. But we can *quicken* the pace and climb swiftly by taking ourselves in hand, *by training the mind*.

The mind is a queer storehouse. The school-boy bakes his brain on a dry course of lessons daily. Why? To train the mind. That is education: Controlling the well-nigh uncontrollable: the ever-moving, ever-vibrating mind.

We read a good deal and all to no purpose. Dry learning never brings peace of mind. It never gives control over the mind. It never develops the *will*, nor does it unfold the consciousness. It simply leads to brain-fag; *mental cramp*.

Diffusion of thoughts leads to confusion of results. Now suppose the brain to be a road filled with mud. A carriage rolls down the road. The wheels have left a deep, straight track right along the road. Another carriage passes on and *deepens* the track. It is exactly so with the brain. One thought passes through it and a track is made through the grey matter. The intensity of the thought will determine the depth of the track.

As we think, nerve-tracks are created and the repetition of the same thought deepens that nerve-track. New sets of atoms start into activity. Brain-cells are multiplied, and fresh layers of matter cover up these tracks. A similar thought gives them a blow and they are *shaken up*, as it were, into new life.

Reading conveys suggestions to the brain and *induces* certain trains of thought. The human will, if it presses a thought with vigor, increases in force and mental electricity is thus generated. This is "*thought-force*" in a nutshell.

Now far greater pressure is exerted if we think by ourselves. The fine nerves of the brain put themselves in a state of tension, more life flows into them, and, as this goes on, the inner powers of consciousness, of which the brain is only an instrument, are called forth from their potential into an *active, vigorous* condition.

We should read only those books which yield us fresh strong thoughts, *in a line with* our own aims and aspirations in life. People take up a book and start reading page after page with the speed of an express train. The mind is in a state of utter confusion and but faint impressions are being made. *This is most foolish*. Haste makes waste, remember!

Books contain thoughts. If these thoughts are *clean, pure, uplifting, stimulating*, and *instructive* in nature, we should pause upon them and *suck* all the life out of them.

Let a student sit down to read. Let him read a sentence slowly; then let him try to grasp the thought, and think it over intently. *One thought suggests other thoughts*. Thus let him think; stretch his imagination in connection with that thought as far as possible, and drop it only when he has found a clear-cut, distinct conclusion. Let him thus continue for *fifteen teen minutes*. He will possibly feel quite tired at the end. But as he continues the practice of deliberate thinking, he will feel a new assurance of power awakening in his mind. "Read for five minutes; think for ten"—there you have the whole secret.

The above practice is very easy, yet most valuable. It will expand your brain and unfold your Higher Consciousness.

The fact is there is too little manhood in men. Earnestness of the right sort is conspicuous by its absence. Such things as *spiritual Unfoldment—the conquest of self*, are striven after by but few men. Hence when they resolve upon achieving these, the initial difficulties quench their ardour.

First of all we must idealise these Higher Teachings, if we have not done so in the past. We must love them as the *only* things worthy of achievement. It is not the passion of selfish growth that should grip us, but the clear, cheerful atmosphere of purity that should be our guide.

Then when the thoughts of mind are strung up to action we should find nothing difficult of achievement.

Come day, go day, we must stick to our resolve like grim death. *Nothing can crush the spirit*, when it has learned to *recognise* itself.

Hence let us *cherish, nourish*, and *embellish* our Higher Nature by taking upon our shoulder a little of the heavy Karma of the world. Let us do all that we can for our growth, but let us remember that selfishness when it develops is "like a serpent that warms to life by the heat of our hands." Do not then nurse this viper in your bosom. Be as helpful as you can.

MAN: ANIMAL AND DIVINE

BY the side of the Ganges, close to the Desaswamedh Ghat, there sits a man of nearly seventy. He is stark naked. Clad in nature's own garb, the Paramahamsa remains seated in one place, morning, noon and night.

Look at his face. He is of fair complexion. His forehead rises dome-like above his eyes which are clear, serene, and brilliant with soul-fire. His lips have a firm set. In short, his calm and thoughtful eyes, noble forehead, and general features indicate unruffled calmness, great self-control, and immense will-power.

For more than eight years he has been there. In the burning mid-day sun of June, when the very ground seems all a-fire, in the biting, bitter cold of December, he sits there. People flock to him in hundreds daily, bring food enough to fill at least thirty stomachs, bow to him, and tell him their many griefs. All his reply is a nod of his head and a look from his eyes. He eats a few fruits and drinks a little milk, and the rest of the food he scatters among people ever ready to pick it up. He never talks, never laughs or even smiles. His face is always solemn, calm and rapt. If you go near him as I did, you *feel his presence* at once. It is at once a magnetic, powerful, and an all-round spiritual personality.

Now just turn from this Yogi,—for he is nothing else—and follow me to the fish-market. I have been there only once, but I will tell you something about it.

It was eight o'clock in the morning. No less than five hundred men, women and boys were there. My first feeling was one of extreme nausea. (There was a strong, dirty, abominable smell about the place.) The fisher-men had brought in fine, living, leaping fish in their nets. They started by taking these out and beating each *living* fish dead against the hard, brick floor of the market. Squabbling, haggling, abusing, spitting were in full swing. *The evil stink was nothing to them*. It was the smell of the rose-flower, as it were. I went out; rather, *ran out*.

I saw many men and women coming out, their hands full of the dirty stuff. Young men, within their teens, were there. Their eyes were pale and hollow, their skins hung loose upon their bones; their faces denoted greed and lust. I saw not one person who had a healthy, steady, self-reliant look; they seemed like a pack of beggars who had stumbled into a little money which they must spend upon fish.

Indeed, how can it be otherwise? Now comparing one of these back-boneless men with the Saint, what conclusion do you draw?

The one is the ANIMAL-MAN, the other, the DIVINE-MAN.

In the one Fear, Greed, Lust, Superstition have made their home. *The horrors of the slaughter-house do not shock him at all.* His fleshy coating reflects the inner man out and out. His senses are gross and coarse-fibred.

In the other, God is manifesting Himself. He is proof against the extreme heat and cold, lust and passion. If a thunder-bolt were to fall upon him, he would not lose his calmness even for the fraction of a moment.

Is not that real happiness? To realise that you are not the body; that you can never die; that nothing can touch you; that fire cannot burn you; the sword cannot pierce you, the water cannot drown you; to realise your independence of and mastery over the flesh.

This is the true mission of religion. *Religion is being and becoming*. It is not talk. It is not intellectualism. It is not worldism. It is Life and Love.

"God is Love." Love is unselfish. It burns for everyone. It does not come *easily*. Only when we have suffered much, thought much, then and then alone gleams of this Universal Love shine upon us. *It is the dawn of divinity—Spiritual Awakening*.

A time comes when we feel this truth, and sympathy for the sufferings of others is the first sign. *To serve others is a high privilege*. God grants us this opportunity for cleansing ourselves; no higher step can be taken unless we have learnt to be selfless in service.

Happiness is not the goal of life, nor is enjoyment. Those that hunt for it never get it. God is the goal of life. Realising Him we realise happiness.

"Such is the power of good that even the least done brings the greatest results."

Obey God, serve men. Before you have gone far in this vast path, peace will fold its wings around you. Fear will drop away. Worry will be known no more.

Therefore train yourself to serve others, if only one soul. If you have a father, a mother, or some one else depending upon you, serve them with whole-hearted zeal. Care not for gratitude, friend;—*that is their business*. If you are in earnest—*and the mere fact of your reading Yoga proves that you are on the Higher Path*—you will *force* yourself to be unselfish. In a short time your Higher Nature will assert itself and it will become your second Nature.

Let us learn to forget our troubles as soon as possible, for these are not permanent.

"Shattered be Self, Life and Hope. I will try my humble best to help others with body, brain, and soul;" let that be your brave cry. I am with you in this and so are thousands of others.

Each man is a channel for the expression of God's truths. As we evolve from within outwards we conform ourselves to the reception of certain gifts. Each man is a power in himself. We have to rise to our best each time we call truths out. They exist in us potentially and are ever seeking an outlet for right expression.

It rests with us entirely what and how far we will unfold. Fate follows us only so long as we fly from it.

Contact with a stronger mind, a purer heart, is decidedly to our advantage. It acts as a push upwards. You may be poor in riches, but you may be rich in God's greatest gift—purity in word, deed and thought.

You are as great as any one, mark you. Daily you have to light the Lamp of Light Eternal in the secret chamber of your heart. *Right knowledge with its right exercise* will wipe out your misery, which is ignorance—the greatest enemy of man. Remember, knowledge is within you and never outside.

Let me advise you to read sacred things and then *reflect upon* them. Study the feelings and thoughts that arise within you. Leave the faults of others alone. Look upwards but never look down upon your inferiors.

If you study and meditate, if you analyse yourself honestly, you shall surely bury all your weakness in the Light of knowledge. You will rise to the highest level of godliness in time.

LIVE UP TO IT. If you fail, rise again, and again and yet again. Assert yourself; and strength will surely come.

Sincere in your wish, strong in your resolve, nothing can stand in your path. Once again I say *Look ever upwards and onwards.*

DOUBLE CONSCIOUSNESS

THE ancients had a most significant concept as to the intellectual make-up of Man, and before we proceed with our personal remarks on this topic, we shall try to give our readers just a passing glimpse of their view point. Says Aristotle: "There are in the fact of our knowledge two elements analogous to matter and form i.e., a passive principle and an active principle; in other words, there are two kinds of Intellect, the one material or passive and the other formal or active, the one capable of becoming all things by thinking on them, the other making things intelligible. That which acts is necessarily superior to that which suffers; consequently that active intellect is superior to the potential one. The active intellect is separate, impassable and imperishable; the passive intellect on the contrary is perishable and cannot do without the active intellect. Therefore the veritable intellect is the *Separate Intellect* and this intellect alone is eternal and immortal." Dr. Nishikanta commenting on this passage, says: "The function of this passive intellect is to receive all the data of sensation and that of the *Active Intellect* is to collect and compare, and by analysis and synthesis to raise those sensuous or sensorious data to ideas and conceptions."

Now, I suppose, I might explain it in the light of modern psychology somewhat in this way: The senses, namely, touch, taste, smell, sight and hearing, together with the nervous systems, form the various lines of communication between the *Ego* and the *non-ego*, between the *Self* and the *not-self*, between *purusha*—to use the technicality of our Sankaya Philosophy—and *Prakriti*. The plastic mind of the child, like the photographer's sensitized plate is exposed to stimuli from the external world. Impressions from outside—the environmental conditions, i.e., the times, circumstances, and various other surrounding influences—impinge upon the mind and various combinations of brain-cells are formed. Registrations are enforced by further and further combinations, and the continued influx of impressions tend to the definite shaping of these brain-cells, according as one set of impressions *corresponds* with another and so on, till, in time, varying sets of group-cells are formed resulting in habits. The sum total of these impressions establishes itself in the mind of the child as tastes, likes and dislikes, inclinations and predilections. Their relative merits or demerits must be traced to the moulding influence of the early impressions. The child with the widening of its knowledge distinguishes between pleasurable and painful impressions. The child with the painful impressions, connects past with present, rejects painful impressions, accepts pleasurable ones and thus learning to identify impressions by repetition, develops memory. Thus sensation produced thought; for, "Mind, as we know it, is resolvable into states of consciousness, of varying duration, intensity, complexity, etc., all, in the ultimate, resting on Sensation" (Secret Doctrine). The repetition of vibrations, by attraction and repulsion to pleasurable and painful sensations developed memory. The contemplation of the images mirrored in the mind produced knowledge, discrimination and reason; the desire to change from one state to another led to the manifestation of *Will* or energy, the inter-play of thought and desire gave birth to emotion.

Thus, however crudely put, we may for the nonce take it that the concrete mind with the physical brain as its organic base of operation is the *passive intellect* transmitting sensations to the thinker, who reasons upon same in his own sphere and who hence forms the centre of the *Active Intellect*. The passive mind is so much matter appropriated from the not-self, for certain purposes. It is alive or seems so because the ego works in and through it. Averros, the great commentator on Aristotle has made it all very clear: "The Passive Intellect aspires to unite with the Active Intellect as the potential calls for the Actual, as the matter calls for the form, or as the flame rushes for the combustible body. But the effect is not confined to the first degree of possession only, called the acquired intellect. The Soul can arrive at a much more intimate union with the universal intellect at a sort of identification, with *Primordial Reason*. The acquired intellect has served to lead man up to the sanctuary but it disappears as that object has been gained, very nearly as sensation prepares the way for imagination and disappears as soon as the act of Imagination is too intense. In this way, the active intelligence exercises on the soul two distinct influences, of which the one has for its object, to elevate the material or passive intellect to a perception of Intelligibles, while that of the other is to draw it further up to a union with the Intelligibles themselves. Arrived at this state man understands all things by the Reason he appropriated to himself. Having become similar to God, he is in a certain sense all the beings that exist and knows them as they really are; because the being and their causes are nothing beyond the knowledge that he possesses of them. There is in every being a tendency to receive as much of this finality as suits his nature. Even the animal shares it and bears in itself the potentiality of arriving at this

Being." The Higher Mind or the Active Intellect in each individual is a ray from the *Universal Mind* and since that is the common source, all minds are resolvable into *One Mind:*—the varying types of mentality between man and man being really due to changing cycles of race-evolution in varying environments.

SPIRITUAL UNFOLDMENT

THE heart of man pants for many things. *Desire moves man more than aught else.* Passions may lash up the lake of his mind into a thousand pulsations; grief may burn the iron of despair right into his brain, and make him feel as one stranded; all his emotions and feelings may play upon him; the world outside may fasten its grip upon him, toss him up from pillar to post and beat him flat; yet the impress left by these is sooner or later wiped out and man rises to his feet once more. But not so the iron grip of desire. It holds on to him like grim death. It drags out the soul minute after minute of our existence, electrifies the unwilling hand to exertion and stimulates the brain to accomplish its ends.

From the hoary, venerable sage, standing triumphant upon the heights of spirituality, down to the most animalized, coarsened man—the Bushman, the Central African savage—this phenomenon makes itself clearly visible to the observant eye.

Now, there come moments in our lives, when even the greatest money-spinners; the most persistent pleasure-hunters, turn aside from their usual occupations to listen to a *voice* within them which is constantly asking, *"Man, where art thou from? Where art thou drifting along? To what end is all this?—Money, wife, children, and all that you hold next to your heart.* "What has a man gained, if he has gained the whole world and lost his soul?"

These and similar other questions beat upon our brains in spite of all our contrary partialities, our thorough worldism.

All this unrest and discomfort *is quite in the nature of things*. Man cannot always be building mud-pies and swallowing "goldpills." Something more abiding, more permanent, is wanted. This yearning after the Eternal makes us call a halt upon the pursuit of blind passions, the hunt after pleasure,— which is the vanishing point between satiety and reaction.

The son wants to be united to the Father, his primal source. God becomes an indispensable necessity. Without Him, life seems to be a dance after fleeting shadows. Each word of advice, of guidance and of spiritual help comes as a cup of cold water to the thirsting soul.

Life is simplicity itself. *It is governed everywhere by One Life, One Law, One Word*,—such is the grand teaching of the Ancients. And as we, by knowledge, experience and observation, get a clearer grasp of this doctrine of *Unity*, we approach *Truth*.

As our vision of God grows more and more distinct, Life with its million, million tongues, seems all music. Fear is sloughed off like a dead skin. Peace, poise and power are all attracted to us by the subtle magnetism of pure thoughts. Man eyes man with Love, Compassion and Pity. The fibres of the mind have grown too finely strung to stand the shock of evil thoughts and desires, and *these latter* fly off from the keenly vibrant mind. Listen to Yogi Ramacharaka:

"From this point you will gradually develop into that consciousness which assures you that when you say "I" you do not speak of the individual entity with all its power and strength but know that the "I" has behind it the power and strength of the spirit and is connected with an inexhaustible supply of force, which may be drawn upon when needed. Such an one can never experience Fear—for he has risen far above it. Fear is the manifestation of weakness and, so long as we hug it to us and make a bosom friend of it, we will be open to the influence of others. *But by casting aside Fear we take several steps upwards in the scale. . . . When man learns that nothing can really harm him, Fear seems a folly*. And when man awakens to a realisation of his real nature and destiny, he knows that nothing can harm him and consequently Fear is discarded.

"It has been well said, "There is nothing to fear but fear." . . . The abolition of Fear places in the hands of man a weapon of defence and power which renders him almost invincible. Why do you not take this gift which is so freely offered you? *Let your watchwords be "I am;" "I am fearless and free."*

The italics are mine. It is a lengthy quotation but each word will repay perusal.

Thus we see that "Spiritual Unfoldment" means a gradual stripping off of the dense and subtle sheaths in which man is clothed for the manifestation of the spirit.

What is the Spirit? I can give you but a very poor idea. The spirit is the highest principle, the most sublime attribute of Man. According to the teachings of advanced occultists and the great sages of India. *Man is a sevenfold creature; is also in seven sheaths;* manifests on seven planes of being.

These are according to Yogi Ramacharaka's classification: 7 Spirit; 6 Spiritual mind; 5 Intellect; 4 Instinctive Mind; 3 Prana, Vital Force; 2 Astral Body; 1 physical body.

Few, almost none of the present race, have achieved the seventh principle. The spirit in man is a spark from the Divine Flame. It establishes a psychic connection, if I may so put it, between Man and the Absolute. The noblest of men, the most wonderful geniuses, the most brilliant master-minds, were the fortunate recipients of a few flashes of the spirit, which is the Invincible Controlling Power in Man. In moments of deep abstraction, the human consciousness, if concentrated upon high ends, finds messages from the Spirit flash downwards, like a streak of lightning; and the world is startled by the revelation.

As I have remarked before, Man is not a finished product of nature. He is a developing creature. He has to *master* all these sheaths and realise the spirit within—*Himself*.

It is a long and serious task. Those that take it up consciously, undertake the most trying task of life. Yet we are all going that way.

Here are three words:—*Instinct, Reason, Intuition*. These are the three phases of mind, from the lowest up to the highest. They develop into each other. Instinct dovetails into Reason, and Reason into Intuition. Let us consider them categorically.

The instinct is a subconscious intelligence. There is a *self-preserving principle* of the mind. The animal world illustrates this. One animal fights another, kills another, to maintain its life. The duckling rushes to the water as its natural element; the newly-fledged bird wants to be on the wing; the child seeks the mother's breast as its source of nourishment; our feet run away with us in moments of peril in spite of ourselves;—*it is all Instinct*. The various work of the body, digestion, assimilation, tissue change, etc., are all carried on along this subconscious line of mentation. Passion is said to be *blind*, because it is a part of the Instinct.

This lowest phase of the mind is most developed in man. It has no reason, no volition.

As man grows, he begins to think, to compare himself with others, to analyse things, to classify, to judge, and so on. This is Reason. It is the Intellect, with the conscious entity, "I" as its monarch. The baby ego, the hitherto sleeping soul, begins to wake up at its magic touch. *The will becomes rationalized*. It shows itself *by assertions, demands and commands*.

Through the intellect man learns to recognize his developing manhood. His self-consciousness, the "*I am*" consciousness, expands and learns to regard himself as a distinct, living, reasoning being.

The intellect controls the Instinctive mind. It checks it from picking up suggestions dropped by others. The will as it develops swings brain and body, the "lust of the flesh, the lust of the eyes, the pride of life" round to its own mandates. The half developed intellect is a source of misery. It sends fear thoughts, adverse suggestions, into the Instinctive Mind, which, slave-like, carries out orders blindly.

Into the Intellect, when it has touched its zenith shades the Spiritual Mind, Intuition. Intuition passes beyond, transcends the intellect. It is the "Super-conscious Mind." All that is considered noble and lofty in the mind comes from the spiritual mind. The "brotherhood" of man and the "fatherhood" of God: "True religious feelings, kindness, humanity, justice, unselfish love, mercy, sympathy, etc., come to us through slowly unfolding spiritual mind"

Intuition is the highest phase of the human mind. it sees truth by direct perception. It is the seat of prophesy, inspiration and spiritual insight. As the mind becomes calm and controlled, rays of light penetrate it from the realms of the spirit. Prophesy, the intuitive perception of some future event, often shows itself. It is a faculty which belongs to the spiritual side of consciousness. It is superior to our physical, astral and mental selves. It transcends the human and shades into the Divine.

Such, in brief, is a crude conception of Spiritual Unfoldment. It does scant justice to this subject, yet it may go to throw some light on some dark problems.

Man is not a sack of flesh, blood and bones. We are all of us traveling Godwards. We have not been born to dance to the orders of others; nor is enjoyment the aim of. life.

Some people, who have developed a little intellect, regard themselves as the *créme de la créme* of the universe. "We are in a higher sphere." Such is the blindness of conceit. Those that cultivate such ideas will find the ground cut from under their feet.

Let us pick out our line of action carefully. Let us not go into society an Ishmael with our hand raised against every one. Selfish, grasping men are the most unhappy of the whole lot of us. *Harm watch, harm catch*.

None of us are spotless. If there is any one who repels us, let us not hate him. *There is nothing to hate but hatred*.

Wisdom and an understanding of our place in the vast cosmic Evolution alone can rob Death of its terrors.

The warm, living impulses of the heart, if carried out, will surely work for our upliftment. Religion is life. Its mission is to take the *animal-man* out of the *divine-man* and set us free from this cage of flesh.

CAUSE AND EFFECT

BY your great enemy I mean yourself. If you have the power to face your Own Soul in the darkness and silence, you will have conquered the physical or Animal-Self that dwells in sensation only."—"*Light on the Path.*"

The above sentence embodies in a nutshell the very cream of the Yoga Philosophy. It is the quintessence of Occultism. 'The lips of wisdom are closed except to the ears of understanding.' You who read this will profit thereby only if you are bent upon *spiritualising* yourself. The One Thing that I want of you is EARNESTNESS: not the earnestness of a-small-pot-soon-hot style, but one deep, abiding and constant impulsion that shall compel your being right through life. There is a widespread impression amongst those of the West that the Yogi is fit only for the lunatic asylum. But before you so clap them into Bedlam, please read, mark, and inwardly digest this lesson and judge it on its merits alone. "Never utter these words 'I do not know this thing, therefore it is not true.' One must study to know, know to understand, and understand to judge." The man whose thoughts are matter-bound, is treading upon beds of quicksand. He is sitting upon a mine that may explode any moment. The only safe course is the Life of the Spirit. Those that lead this life seem to live and breathe in quite a different sphere. They are the true Yogis; the first fruits of humanity. In matters of Self-discipline they neither spare themselves nor others that would learn at their feet. To those moles that are still burrowing into the mud their methods, ever drastic, appear far-fetched. But this is emphatically not so. The Yogi is thoroughly *rational*. He has a profound intellect. He is the picture of health. He is full of kindness and pity. He is ever self-sacrificing, ever *strong* and as to *chastity, he is the very embodiment of it*;—he simply radiates purity. Wherever the Yogi goes he seems to cleanse the very atmosphere of the place by his mere presence. He is calm, serene, and even-minded. He has almost superhuman self-control. In the moment of action, he is the man of cool nerves, of level head, and great penetrating concentration.

One mental scientist in America puts health upon the heights. Why? Simply because there are fifty millions there who are disease-ridden and many a suffering one is a *Moriturus* i.e., at the point of death. This is the result of *materialism*. The gods have put their ban upon it. "Seek ye the kingdom of heaven and all else shall be added unto thee." This is the tremendous advice of the Supreme Master.

The higher life is the only life that is worth living. All else is mere touch-and-go. Now one great secret of success was enunciated by a perfect Yogi. It is the greatest I know. I am fully convinced of its potent force. Let me give it to you:

Join the means to the end, and you have the sum-total; the objective; the goal that you are striving for and aiming at. The result is in direct ratio to the intensity of the effort. The greater the effort, the greater the result. There is an ever-continuing, never-slackening tension of this spiritual law of *cause* and *effect*, of *sowing* and *reaping*. We only get what we deserve;—not an iota more or less. The gods hold the scales evenly and Nature deals in even-handed justice. No honest seeking ever goes unrewarded. We have to perfect the means. We have to adjust efforts to obstacles. If the action is incoordinate, so shall be the result. Give and it shall be given unto you. Everything is in a circle. *What we do, that we have*. In taking all possible care of the means, you are simply starting currents of force into activity. These must complete the circuit and come back to you, the centre, in time. Therefore what we have to do is to work, work, and work. The results cannot but come. Your body is so constituted that it renews itself after each exertion; with each fresh effort, there is a corresponding inrush of force. He who works his hardest, has the most energy. Energy is ever withdrawn from those that would spend same with a niggardly hand. *The supply is exactly in proportion to the exhaust*. It is the pressure at which we live that counts most. Life is unnecessarily long;—only, so much time we spend in vegetating rather than living. For only the spiritual man can appreciate the fine art of living. As a great thinker said: We ask for long life, but 'tis deep life, or grand moments, that signify. Life culminates and concentrates. Homer said "The gods ever give to mortals their appointed share of reason only on one day."

"Just to fill the hour—that is happiness. Fill my hour ye gods, so that I shall not say, 'whilst I have done this, Behold, also an hour of my life is gone,' but rather, 'I have lived an hour.'"

"In stripping time of its illusions, in seeking to find what is the heart of the day, we come to the quality of the moment and drop the duration altogether. It is the depth at which we live and not at all the surface extension, that imports. We pierce to the eternity of which time is the fitting surface; and really the least acceleration of thought and the least increase of power of thought, make life to seem and to be of vast duration. *We call it time, but when that acceleration and that deepening effect take place, it acquires another higher name;*—ETERNITY"

"*God works in moments.*"

"*The measure of life, O Socrates, is with the wise;—the speaking and hearing such discourses as yours.*"

"*There is no real happiness in this life but in intellect and virtue.*"

"It is the deep today that all men scorn, the rich poverty which men hate; the populous, all-loving solitude which men quit for the tattle of towns. He lurks, he hides;—he who is Success, Reality, Joy and Power. One of the illusions is that the present hour is not the critical hour, the decisive moment. Write it on your heart that every day is the best day in the year. No man has learned anything rightly until he knows that every day is Doomsday. 'Tis the oldest secret of the gods that they come in low disguises."

"*Nature shows herself best in leasts.*"

The above are just a few thoughts to convince you that each stroke, each swing of the Will, each moment of utter devotion to the means, each hour of day, uncongenial labor, each spell of painful, patient concentration shall count in the Eternal Summation.

Hence pay homage to and worship the means. Honour the present moment. Set up the strong *Present Tense* against all else. The present moment is the crystalisation of the Past. Build into the structure of the Past the *richest* and *finest* materials, vitalize it with the *rich, red, life-blood of youth*, and surely, most surely, the spirit shall *shine out* in all its *columnar majesty*. Your Past is laden with the *cumulative force of thoughts, desires and actions. Everything turns upon how you have lived in the past.*

How cramped, how down-trodden, how sorrow-laden, how miserable, how low, mean, and hard-hearted and cruel we men and women are!

It all seems to have been *ground* in with our life-force. Stop right *now*, NOW, and examine yourself in the clear light of the intellect. Ten to one, you *shudder* at your hideous weaknesses, that darken and defile your Nature.

"*What I would that I do not; what I would not, that I do.*" "*When I would do good, evil is present with me.*"

This is the tale of the age. It is a staggering blow to one's optimism. It dampens one's spirits. It plunges one into the bottomless pit of despair. Standing by men steeped to their lips in weaknesses, one turns inwards and doubtingly says "Am I really Strong?"

"*I failed.*" Why? "Because, sir, you *neglected* the MEANS and simply killed your time in spinning *airy webs*. You did not throw in your heart and soul. Here is the *cause* and *cure* of failure. In our struggles to cheat Nature, we simply cheat ourselves. In trying to drown the voice of conscience, we simply sink ourselves. In trying to follow the eat-drink-and-be-merry policy we simply RETARD our own *inner unfoldment.*

Please remember therefore:—All Yogis are tremendous *causationists*. *There is method in their madness*. They believe in methodical and persistent work. They say with me in effect:—

"*Marshal your forces properly and powerfully and success is sure.*"

Is it not meet that we turn to something permanent, something that will live through the ages, some-thing that will be a powerful lever to uplift, inspire, and ennoble others?

"*It is! It is!*" that's what you say.

To be able to appreciate greatness at its full value, we must ourselves have the germs of greatness stirring within us. The power of the spirit is struggling to uncoil itself. Your being vibrates to the thrills of spiritual forces. Your complex though confused ideas regarding your mission, your Divine Heritage, your birthright, are shooting into order. The pressure of your chains is telling upon your nerves. Your sufferings, your little independent *twists* and *angles* and *blind gropings* are the promises of your future.

Intensify yourself then along these channels. Carry these thoughts constantly with you. Make them the part, nay, the whole, of your lives. They shall fit in everywhere. *Ever they ring true.* I hear this complaint from many men. "I am deeply impressed when I read these things or when you talk of them to us. I am full of noble resolves. I feel quite different from hum-drum humanity. But alas! the impression wears off as soon as the world demands my attention."

That shows positively that the latter compels your nature. The superficial glamour of worldism claims you for its own as Mephistopheles claimed Faust. Your carnal and sex-sensational tendencies occupy the *"principal seats"* in your nature. Your talk of the Higher Life is vapory in the extreme; you are like Clarence Glyndon in Lytton's "Zanoni:"—"Unsustained Aspiration" *would follow instinct, but is deterred by conventionalism—is overawed by idealism, yet attracted and transiently inspired; but has not steadiness for the initiatory contemplation of the Actual. He conjoins its snatched privileges with a besetting sensualism and suffers at once from the horror of the one and the disgust, involving the Innocent (others) in the fatal conflict of his spirit:*" (Mirror of young manhood.)

MAN—THE MASTER

MEN are going up an ascending scale of existence. Some have their feet still planted upon the lowest rungs of the ladder. Others have climbed higher and higher.

At the start, the functions of life are all performed upon a semiconscious plane. The law of life is for progress, struggle, achievement and realization. The force of this law swings the physical and mental mechanism of Man to its own beneficent purpose and propels them to action. Progress at this stage is on the sub-conscious plane of mentation.

The soul is in a comatose condition. Impacts from the physical world, the driving power of the lave of Progress—Evolution,—and the inherent powers of the soul, all combine to push us on.

Man's central Being is *infinite bliss*. I am Happiness itself. I am unhappy because my eyes have grown blind.

Yes, Man has forgotten his real, divine Nature. Cycle after cycle of activity thus goes on. Man is being worked upon by a Divine Law whose stern mandate is "*Awake, Arise, and Stop not till the goal is reached*."

Not all of us hear it thus. The pious Christian devoutly believes, "Oh, There is an Evil Force, Satan, whose arm strikes me down. Good Lord, Thou alone art my refuge."

In praying thus he believes in the Infinite power of the absolute; and since nothing is lost in the economy of Nature, he delivers a concentrated suggestion to his soul, which alone is Infinite. He believes that his prayer will bear fruit, and it does. In believing he delivers the right blow and his belief is fulfilled.

It is a very good thing to pray; to believe that Providence is always playing with your destiny, to believe that a mighty Mephistopheles is laying traps for you, to believe that the body dying, the soul does not die, to believe that God alone can save you.

The good side of it lies in your repulsion of Evil. Fear and at times love of the Infinite make you cleave to good.

But do not stop there. Your attitude is out and out a negative one. You cannot always stand by your none-too-well-grounded convictions. Facts go to prove this. In this world you often see a man born in poverty, squalor and sin. He has not a single chance in life. Then take a man born to the purple. There is nothing to vex him. Plenty stalks majestically in the land. He has but to wish and to! it is fulfilled.

"Everything that God commands is for the best," you say. "Perhaps his father is to blame," some one would say.

First, why should I be punished for the sins of my father, secondly why should I not be created as my friend is? Why should every one laugh at my Physical, Mental and Spiritual endowments; how do I deserve this?

"God's ways are inexplicable," you say. Very fine, indeed!

Friend, God does not love mystery mongering. He can never give us pain without rhyme or reason. My experience tells a different tale. God is Love. He acts in open daylight. We go to Church and say long prayers for sins committed. We shall commit that same sin again and again; and we shall cease only when repeated blows rub the lesson home. "You must cease from this. It has back of it the most painful results."

Man is punished not for his sins so much as by them. Nature with her pitiless ways cannot claim mercy for herself. Her laws are hard. Be it a sin of commission or of omission, your escape is impossible. This penalty bears a mission peculiar to itself. Ili is a blessing in disguise. It is the merciful knife of the surgeon. If there is loss, pain, suffering, disappointment at one pole, it is all counterpoised by the ripening of experience, wisdom, knowledge at the other. Hence measured on the scale of Compensation, all pain, come it how it may, must be faced with patience. Pain comes in jangled vibrations, seems to asphyxiate the whole man, strikes us down for the needed lesson. In suffering we pay our debts. The burden is lightened. Sin and suffering are twins and separation is impossible. How we wish we had been let off scot-free; how like miserable shirkers we wish our bed had no crumpled rose leaves. Yet would you who weep and lament be minus the experience and wisdom you have stored up through efforts to brush pain aside? No right have we then to rule off pain as a visitation of a wrathful Deity. Rather, we shall see Cause and Effect, not somewhere and sometimes but everywhere and always. That is the position of Strength. Every sweet has its sour. We shall confront fate with fate, fire with fire, and, standing aside, see the one eat the other. The end of all philosophy is the destruction of pain. Not milksops and lunatics, but men of iron courage are philosophers. Philosophy is thought passed and purified through the fire of the Living Spirit. It is deathless, birthless truth established in the constitution of man. Clay and clay differ, they say, so thought and thought vary in power, tenacity and texture. Man is a living magnet. He attracts. He repels. He draws in his own; he throws out what is not related to him. As Emerson, the western child of eastern thought sings:—

> 'And all that Nature made thy own,
> Floating in air or pent in stone
> Will rive the hills and swim the sea,
> And, like thy shadow, follow thee.'

Just that comes to us which is ours by right of thought; just that flies off from us which is not ours, What we seek we shall find; what we flee from, will flee from us; as Goethe said, "What we wish for in youth comes to us in heaps in old age." Everything on the zone of our mental vibration will be ours. Remember you who read! Thought is a mighty force. It is your friend. It is your enemy. As your ideal in life, along that line will Everything flow. You are a Spark from the Eternal Fire and as is proved in Higher Mathematics *the parts of Infinity are an Infinity; you too are Infinite*. God re-Exists in each mortal form. His light shines full upon your Consciousness. You wish, you command, you demand, you assent, and you get—what you want; though you go to sleep, your thought if sufficiently vitalized by concentration will come to pass. Determine the breadth, the solidity, the soundness of the plank of life you stand upon. You are your master. Knowing and realizing this, you shall step up to the highest and best in life and with firm hands pluck the fruit you would taste. The sweet, the bitter, or the bittersweet taste is according as you choose. Where and what is *Fear* then? It is all cause and effect. Laugh at Astrology, at Palmistry; know their secrets; know they are emanations from you; and stand fearless and strike straight from the shoulders, once, twice, thrice, times innumerable till your strokes tell, till your strokes lay low the monsters that have broken their teeth upon your unyielding shoulders; till you have what you should have. *This, friend, is a passing glimpse of Life's Conscious Stage. Here Life is self-determined. Here no hand but yours builds. No brains but yours thinks. No strength but yours avails. No soul but yours bids, bargains and at last bears away the palm.*

SELF-DEVELOPMENT

The Objective Mood.

MAN should ever strive to develop intrinsic worth. Life becomes a song of harmony, Peace and Power, when once you have developed and expanded the Will-power. The education of the Will should be the aim of your life. The pleasure-seeker is an ass. He is ever complaining of his hard lot, of disappointment, of ill-health; he is as a bird bereft of wings, quivering its shattered pinions in its vain attempt to soar up in the sky. He is a leaning willow whose whole structure indicates weakness and dependence. The gods have put their ban upon this twentieth century fever for pleasure. Go into any large assembly of educated men and if you are a true judge of character you will hardly pick out five men out of five hundred with the fine, refined impressive features of Stoic, a heroic soul in an obedient body. The reason is not far to seek. Their chief object is to titillate the nerves of sensation. They never learned the great and important law of Self denial. They are being dragged along by a force far mightier than their feeble selves. They have never said a firm *No*, to their impulses. They are mere *masks* and not men. They are automatic machines. They may have picked up a little odd knowledge; they may have a law cunning, but they lack the Affirmative Force of Character, the vim and pith of a Positive Personality, the calm poise of controlled energy. They have never realized the intense joy of a soul that lives only to aspire after what is high and noble. But then Existence is not all a bed of roses. Shocks will come and, when they do, these weaklings are bowled over like so many nine-pins. Then they just sit up and talk of their aching hearts, their bleeding wounds, their sorrow laden, miserable lives. Their good wishes are as so many soap-bubbles. Their resolutions are mere effervescence of a dying vitality. Their promises the mere ebullitions of emotion *minus* the stamina to accomplish them. They are the blind worms of fate. They are the victims of wicked-minded men. They are so many will-less, nerve-less weaklings. They are slaves.

Why?

Because, they are in the clutches of Ignorance. Ignorance consists in seeking enjoyment of the senses. To burst the chains that hold you captive, give up, once for ever, the desire To ENJOY, and DETERMINE to positivize the Will-Force for the free and smooth-working of the wheels of Progress, upon which weakness is a clog and must be removed in order to ensure easy action. A man, nearly ten years my senior in age and the father of three children was suffering from dyspepsia. It had become chronic. His was a purely nervous trouble. He was sorely afraid that his stomach had lost all power to digest food. For months he had been ailing. The doctors could give no aid. His fear was always realized. At last after quite three months of painful suffering he one evening came to me. "Can you do anything for me?" "Not knowing the trouble I cannot prescribe the cure;" I replied. "But what am I to do? I shall be a wreck in a short time." "Look here, you are thoroughly mistaken. You fear, and your fear is realized. Fear is a suggestion for adverse conditions. Don't be afraid and everything will be all right. Trust nature; she will do her work." "But how can I master this fear? It paralyzes me and my mind." "Very good," I replied energetically. "Will you obey me?" "Yes,"—he said. "Don't touch any food for seven days." He promised. He had never gone without food for seven days. He fasted for just two days. On the third day he felt famishing for food. He must eat. He did eat. The food was digested. It is six months since he had this trouble and from that time till now he eats freely and digests freely. "When the fear comes over me, I just determine to stop eating and that drives away my fear," he said. The psychological explanation is simple. His determination to stop eating was an antidote to his fear; the former was a Positive Denial of the power of the latter to overcome this man and it scattered the force of Fear.

By evident analogy you can conclude that the mere determination to kill out the desire for enjoyment will bring about a tremendous change of thought-habit and crush your weakness. "If thy right eye offend thee, pluck it out." However keen your suffering you must determinedly pluck out of your nature everything that weakens you. Rest assured, this step, desperate as it is, shall ever strengthen you and, although for the moment you may suffer the torments of Hell, your path shall open out freely. Do not yield. Do not care for life. Die, if need be, but die a strong man that refused utterly to yield to illness. Your flesh may not be able to stand the strain of such action; but your spirit shall live and grow stronger. However, except in extremely desperate cases, the flesh ever helps the spirit when the latter is strong and the body and the life forces at once become the best possible co-operators with their master. Hence determine to stand guard by your High Nature. Draw the line between your animal and your Divine Nature. Cleave to the latter, happen what may. Remember, my readers, Doing alone teaches Doing. Therefore determine to perform your duties according to the dictates of your inner Nature, your conscience, your intuitive Nature. This is the Objective Mood, Doing and not Dreaming. You shall be at the top of your condition if you ever obey the suggestions of your soul, for your heart shall never tell a lie although your tongue may. Determine to be master of your mind and work at this Concentration exercise daily with earnest and hopeful steadfastness; sit up at night in perfect silence. Hold yourself steady bodily and mentally. Then begin to tense your Will. Feel and say "I am this very moment mastering my mind. Now. This moment. Now. Insist on immediate mastery. Do not say "tomorrow," but say "This moment." Set up the strong Present Tense against all else. Do not give up till you are quite exhausted mentally. Do it with perseverance. It will set up strong vibrations that will destroy the weak atoms of your brain and thoroughly establish a vigorous tone of thought-activity. Practice will bring light. Inspiration comes on the vibratory wires of strong thought and strong action. Action, muscular exertion, will tune your mind to a responsive condition, will clinch your intentions into strength and motive power to your entire Nature. Learn to tense your Will. Learn to be positive to evil suggestions, either from your own Nature or from that of others. Have a Spirit of your own. Determine to do a thing and do not desist while there is even a breath left in the body. Greatness could never be a prize for cowards. Only the brave, the pure, the strong, the determined, can reach the goal. None else, none else.

DEVELOPING THE SPIRITUAL CONSCIOUSNESS

"The mind which follows the rambling senses, makes the Soul as helpless as the boat which the wind leads astray upon the waters."
Bhagavad Gita.

MAN is man by virtue of *willing*, not by virtue of knowing and understanding. As he is, so he sees. His hopes and aspirations are in exact proportion to the depth and power of his will: for, says Emerson, "The height of the pinnacle is measured by the breadth of the base."

He is the microcosm of the macrocosm: the little world of the big world. *The universe exists for the self:*—such is the dictum of the sages.

Man has appropriated this form, this coat of skin, for the exercise and unfoldment of his Divine Nature. He is *above* Nature, his body is *of* Nature.

Man, *Know Thyself*, was mandate of the Delphic Oracle. All your efforts, your joys and sorrows, your ups and downs, are to this end. You now grasp this thing, soon you drop it; then you grasp that thing; soon you drop it;— Not this, Not that, you say. This is the speech of Negation: neti, neti: Not this, Not this.

You who are Infinite in essence drank deep of the waters of Lethe and falling under the magic spell of Maya, forgot yourself. You have ever since then been identifying yourself with Nature, with your form, the Not-self. You do not see that this body, this brittle casket of clay, is for disintegration, for dissolution. You love it to infatuation. You draw the cruel, merciless knife across the neck of poor, defenseless animals to gratify your lower Nature. This body must live, though I eat burnt flesh, rotten flesh, to keep it alive. Man would eat man, if his digestion did not get upset, thereby. Do not say 'No,' you animalized ignorant soul! *You swallow camels and yet you strain at gnats*. Thus through extreme attachment to your form, have you contracted your soul, hypnotized yourself into a *finite* being. You alone can strip off your limitations and stand in your *Native* splendour once again. To realize this is to realize divinity—is to transcend Nature!

As you learn to control Nature *within* you, so will you control things *outside* of yourself, so shall your great, all-potent will shine out to the universe.

Man's will is God's will. What is of God is God. The Infinite exists, in full stature, in each living, breathing form. *Hence to know yourself is to know God.* You are Bliss Eternal. You, the Infinite, became confined in sheaths of matter. Your real, immortal self shines aloft, but what little was caught up by the physical mechanism of Consciousness, fell senseless under the hypnotic suggestions of Maya. Yet an impulsion from within is pushing you on. This is the Desire to achieve happiness which is a distorted reflection on the physical plane of your own blissful self that is on the spiritual.

It is the natural magnetism of your real self that is drawing you up. *Ends ascend as Nature descends*, said Swedenborg, the Mystic. *All things are in a scale; and begin where we will, ascend and ascend. All things are symbolical; and what we call results are beginnings:* Emerson, on Plato, the philosopher.

So long as you are flung about under the influence of passions your progress will be clogged. The soul is under the thrall of matter, just as a muscular pair of wrists may be loaded with fetters. It is trying to burst the shackles that chain it down. It is passing through a transition stage. Its continued effort to free itself thoroughly and entirely is the promise of the future. Conquest comes. Yes! Conquest comes. I have not read these two words. I do not repeat them to you like a parrot. It has been given to me to *feel* the fact. Do not say "I cannot. It is beyond me;" say "*I can. It is in me.*" So will you conquer.

This ascension of the soul is the development of the Spiritual Consciousness.

It is not intellectualism: nor spiritualism: nor supernaturalism: nor any other ism.

It is the quickening of your evolution on the spiritual plane by the up-keep of *a systematized line of thought activity plus the self-determined exercise of volition.*

It is the polarization of the human life force up to a high pitch of concentrated exercise of the will-power in Man.

The task is not easy of accomplishment. You can achieve it only by dedicating a whole life time to it. It is worth your while. Aim at thoroughness. Take up the suggestions I pass on. Dream them out. Think them out. Act them out.

Your aim is the subjugation of the animal soul. Have no other aim. "When one becomes freed from the bondage of the senses, he transcends all material relations and realizing the inward light regains his knowledge of Himself—this a realization of the truth. It dwells beyond Mortality and Fear."

One thing at a time and that with your entire heart and soul. The ideal you have set up for yourself must absorb the best and the richest forces in you. Introduce the thin end of the wedge. Each stroke shall drive it deeper. Do not scatter your energy. Do not burn your candle at both ends. The secret of success is Concentration. A man may be an omnivorous reader. He is a walking Encyclopaedia. His brain is a Bodleian Library. Yet he has no worth, no intrinsic qualities, that can give him that breadth and depth of dignity that go out of a man possessing inner force of character.

Remember, You are deathless, birthless. You live in the Eternal. One life-span can be but a short one at best. Therefore arrange your forces so that they shall flow in one even continuous stream along one line. The man who has thus lived upon five ideas in one life, will command more than your Jack-of-all-trades-but-master-of-none man ever can. You must stand body and soul, for your ideas, taking up each and quietly working them out in life. This will avoid much friction and ever insure a clear and steady brain.

Education, said Vivekananda, is a *man-making, life-building* assimilation of ideas.

You must then by patient thinking build up an ideal for yourself. This done, give up all dreaming, all castle-building, and start in for the work. Then three things are necessary for effectual work.

The first is earnest, ardent Desire. Your heart is knitted to things of the earth, earthy, by a myriad of tiny threads. To break up the links, a strong, all-impelling force is needed. Desire ardently, longingly, for perfect establishment of chastity in your Consciousness. This keen desire is a *sine-a-qua-non*. Without it you cannot go through the difficulties that bar your way. Clothe yourself in this panoply of power and the shafts of adverse fortune, shall glance off from your strong armour. If you haven't this gift, it shows that your sense of manhood is small. You lack force. The greater the sinner, the greater the saint. A man must have this force or his good intentions will die a natural death. He can neither be a saint nor a sinner. He is *tamasic*; is of a dull, lazy, ease-loving, insipid nature.

But do not lose heart, if you belong to this class of men. You can cultivate this force. There is always a way out. Your imagination is your creative power. Now there is a close association between thought and imagination. Imagination is thought in its full freedom. Therefore to train the desire-nature you must bring thought to bear upon it. Desire cannot train desire. You are helpless within the narrow limits of the desire aspect of the Self. You desire a thing or you do not; that's all.

No. Thought alone can help you here. Says Emerson:—*There is no thought in any mind but it quickly tends to convert itself into a power, and organizes a huge instrumentality of means.*

One thought repeated for days, months and years will become very strongly vitalized. Tremendous will be its telling force. It will go to make or mar your destiny. As the famous axiom goes, "*Allow the thought, and it may lead to a choice, 'carry out the choice, and it will be the act,' repeat the act and it forms the habit; allow the habit and it shapes the character; continue the character, and it fixes the destiny.*"

Thought, then, is the fine cause. Stamp it well upon your mind. It is a tremendous fact. Learn it well, now: now, while you read it.

Picture to yourself, then, the benefits derivable from control of the lower nature.

See how the man, who is chaste in word, deed and thought, is above the din and strife of conflicting passions. He is calm, serene, and self-poised. Having inner control, the control of the outer is an easy affair with him. He does not go about—anxious for recognition. He is master of himself, and therefore of others. His mere presence brings peace to the troubled souls of others. His speech is as a dash of cold water. It makes you sit up and listen. It stimulates you; it uplifts you; it expands you. Nothing is impossible to you. You seem or feel as if you were another being. The chaste man has communicated himself to you in all his fulness and breadth of nature. He has stirred up forces in you of which perhaps you were never before conscious.

See how the chaste man seems to purify the very air he breathes. See how dauntless is the courage that bubbles up from within him.

See how he is idolized by humanity. The mere sight of him puts new life and vigor in others. His power of doing good seems to have an inexhaustible reservoir behind it.

Thus go on picturing to yourself the all-inclusive uses of chastity.

This is the positive process of Visualization; Mental photography.

Now if your case is desperate, one of long standing, take up the negative process.

Picture to yourself the disappointment, the loss of spiritual force, the gloom and the melancholy, that cloy all passion; the swinish, grovelling, aspect of the sensual soul: the consequent exhaustion: the jeer and ridicule of the world: the breaking-down of all your fond hopes: the pitiable poverty-stricken condition of those dependent on you; the disgraceful passage through death into an even more hideous condition of life: the utter degeneration: the shameful existence: the haunting thoughts beyond.

This method is the negative one. It is like the surgeon's knife used to cut out a cancer that threatens life. Desperate diseases require desperate remedies. This process is not advisable, except in otherwise hopeless cases. Rather use the positive method. As you sit up visualizing your ideal day after day, its attraction to you will be truly magnetic. Your heart shall go out to it in all its force. You shall want to embrace the ideal every moment of your life. Energy will come to you. Indeed your complaint then shall be: I have more energy than I can control, more thoughts than I can marshal up for serene action.

Your thoughts have been energized by constant repetition. Now you must learn to dominate them: to command them to stillness: to relax the tension in which your mind is constantly putting itself: to save your brain from giving way under this surcharge of unmarshalled energy; to absolutely vanquish the waves of force that bubble up each time you think of your ideal; for it is intoxication—the irresistible spell of a "fixed idea."

Says Swami Vivekananda: *The organs are the horses, the mind is the reins, the intellect is the charioteer, the soul is the rider, and this body is the chariot. If the horses are very strong and do not obey the reins, if the charioteer, the intellect, does not know how to control the horses, then this chariot will come to grief. But if the horses, i.e., the organs, are well-controlled, if the reins, i.e., the mind, are well held in the hands of the charioteer, i.e., the intellect, the chariot reaches the goal.*

This then is the line of action. Developing the will-force, the second of the three requisites I spoke of. What is the principle of development? *Exercise*. How did Ram Murti develop his splendid physique, that today is the wonder of the world? *Exercise*. How did Vivekananda develop that terrific magnetism that inundated the entire Parliament of Religions at Chicago? *Exercise*. How did Sheridan who once stuttered in his speech, deliver an oration at the famous Impeachment of Warren Hastings that made the Speaker order an adjournment that the House might recover from the effect of the volcanic play of words. *Exercise*. Be convinced, then, My reader! *Exercise is the first, last, and the only condition of growth*. The human will is the grandest culmination of all the complex workings in the realm of Consciousness. Schopenhauer the philosopher puts will a-top of all else in Nature.

It is a grand thing, this human will. Its influence over man is one of compelling, forcing, driving, impelling, overpowering, commanding, demanding. This force is essentially *Masculine*.

I told you something about the desire-force: drawing, pulling, attracting, charming. This is the *Feminine* phase of Mental energy.

When you combine the two, the positive and the negative electrodes in the human brain, your suggestions whether turned in upon your sub-conscious self or projected outward, command an irresistible position; in fact, they influence the imagination, reason, or will of another man in an uncontrolled man: this is what comes through the practice of Concentration. We should learn to make use of both; whether we are suggesting auto-ally or outwardly.

What is *concentration? Holding the mind to a point*. There are two phases of concentration: a lower and a higher. We shall take up the first only. You are not prepared for the second. Only those whose soul-unfoldment is an actualized fact can practice it and they will not need these teachings. They are their own teachers.

Resolve upon the performance of a certain mental work with concentration, say for half an hour at the beginning. Then carry it out. Do it every day, each time prolonging the duration of the exercise. Suppose you cannot find a mental task. Here is one:

First of all "relax" mentally and physically, yet remain alert and steady. Now: Take this virtue: Chastity. Read literature on this subject. That will provide you with the requisite information and supply many missing links. Study it from the physical, mental, and spiritual viewpoints. Then sit up and calmly think out the bearings of the virtue: What it is? How to practice it; its resulting benefit to humanity; its appreciation; its lifting influence; the sense of courage which it gives; its absolute importance in the quickening of your Evolution and so on and on.

Then steady the mind upon this complete shaping of the virtue. Meditate upon it. Dwell upon it. Will determinedly that it shall become established in you: that from the moment you are sitting in this attitude of Concentrated willing, all your forces are being transmitted to Chastity: that the protoplasm of your very physique are becoming sensitive to the fascination of this virtue: that there is a tremendous force being generated right in the centre of your head that shall present an irresistible front to all evil thoughts and tendencies: that your entire nature vibrates to this thought:—*I am Chaste:* that you recoil instinctively from all that may coarsen your finely-strung spiritual fibres: that evil falls off, flies off, from your intensely poised mind: that your Higher consciousness is unfolding: that your intelligence is expanding: that your will is becoming strong, very strong: that your body obeys you: that you have power, force, within you: and that it all is developing. Now. Say "Now"—"this moment" and insist upon immediate mastery. Do this regularly and at the same time every day.

Thus you can will yourself into any state of mind you like. Not in one day or in one week will you obtain control. It will require a hundred sittings or even more. But from the very first sitting a sense of assurance, the consciousness of an internally developing force, shall come to you:—and this if you have been thoroughly earnest over your task. Perseverance and patience you must have. Indeed! to have these is to have everything. There shall come about a step forward in your evolution at each sitting. This is the art of willing. You get it cheap. Do not treat it with indifference. Practice for a fortnight will prove to you conclusively the verity of my remarks. You have been neck-deep in carnalities: it is high time you thought of a change. Be earnest. Be a determined man. Focus upon an idea and stick to it with the bull-dog's tenacity, till you have seen it through to the end. Do not talk of it to others. Never tell others that you are in! training. Sufficient gratification of your vanity shall you have when you have acquired the wished-for object. The praise of the world is not at all necessary to your happiness. The approval of your own soul is quite sufficient. Each man sets his own measure. If you believe that you are uniquely fitted to be a virtuous pure-hearted man, so will the world also. Stick to your own. Do not be a busy body, for then you shall be nobody. Be an earnest thoughtful man. Stand rigidly by your ideal. Do not force it upon others. But do not be forced out of it. Simply be earnest.

> "To your own self be true,
> and it must follow, as the night the day,
> Thou can'st not then be false to any man."

The third requisite is a keen and broad intelligence. You must not go and buy a pig in a poke. You must not drive a nail where it won't go. By steady and much thinking, you shall be able to expand this faculty. Learn to study in the manner taught in Chapter III—"READ AND REFLECT." There you have instructions that you may well utilize. You will be amply repaid for the trouble of re-reading it. Books supply missing-links and give you the loose-end of suggestions which you can work out at leisure. *Read little, think much*. Your intelligence will be nurtured by contact with a pure soul, for purity charges your body with subtle, radiant and powerful forces. "Socrates declares that if some have grown wise by associating with him, no thanks are due to him, but simply whilst they were with him they grew wise and not because of him." This is the secret. The vibrations of a stronger mind impinge upon your receptive consciousness, shake up some of its grossness, and implant seeds that, fructifying in the long run, work for your spiritual upliftment. Associate with good men. Let their thought-magnetism encircle you and exercise its subtle, mysteriously spiritualizing influence upon you. The mere contact will act as a Living Force and awaken your latent powers. It will shed benediction by its mere touch. Spirituality is not intellectual gymnastics.

It is the life; and life alone can convey life. His words shall wring in your ears even when you are far away from him. His glances shall remain with you, stirring, prompting and stimulating you. This is why India's spiritual teachers command the respect of their pupils.

Thus friend! when you have gone through this simple training, your inner spirit shall transmute all things that approach you to the nature of your ideals. Obstructions will be brushed aside. Many of the vexations and tribulations that you may be suffering now shall be smoothed out of your path. As you speak, as you look, as you move about, your inner nature shall flash out of you. It will enter your hands and feet and compel your entire being. Thus by educating yourself shall you set others a good example. Life will he worth living: Death will lose its horrible aspect: love, power, and peace shall flow out of you, and chasten others. Guard it well. Wield it for good purposes alone. You are now for the divine side of things. Your will is law. Let it be strong and guided by Love. That will develop in your nature *Sattvic* or rhythmic qualities. Then shall you find harmony and peace.

WHO CAN BE A YOGI?

TRUTH knows no death; no birth. It is Eternal; has always been, will always be. Time cannot exhaust its force, for it carries its power within itself. Deep in the heart of Truth is hidden an object we all are groping for. It is power. It is power from the Divine side of things. It is this you seek: the power to be good; the power to bring relief and joy to suffering humanity; the power to shake yourself free from the bondage of your lower nature.

Man always seeks to act out his good wishes, his good intentions. He is here. He clings to this, to that, to all. The cup of desire was presented to our lips. We drank it deep. Its subtle force became embedded in the matrix of our being. It runs in our blood. We just watch its constant play, and watching, say: 'Ah! the cup was mixed too strongly.'

Are you then satiated? Are you tired of being tossed about? of being manipulated for the accomplishment of impermanent ends? of being in the grip of Death, Despot, and Devil? of being ridden over roughshod by the forces of Evil? of being a slave to fear, a subject to wear and tear? of being the blindworm of Fate, the puppet of adverse conditions; conditions that cut up your opportunities in life into tiny bits and scatter same to the winds of heaven? of being hungry for the fleshpots of gold and greed? of being in the thrall of Fear, of Worry, of animalism, of worldism the most shallow and painful? In fine, have you had your fill of slavery? WOULD YOU BE WHAT YOU WILL TO BE? Then learn to say with dauntless courage "*I am Master, not somewhere and sometimes, but everywhere and always. I will put my shoulders to the wheel and hew out my own path. My courage is indomitable. My spirit knows no flagging, no defeat, no despair. I am Fearless and Free*"—this you must learn to say with assurance based upon a clear knowledge of the conditions of your existence; existence not outer, but inner; your inner existence, mark you.

That knowledge is self knowledge. No idle boast of the tongue it is to say with utter conviction "I am Master." Your tremendous assertion must be the outcome of knowledge of the Supreme, of austerities, of purity, of love.

It must be grounded upon experience; and here are a few suggestions just to put you upon the right path.

Man's nature, like all else in Nature, is bi-polar: it is centrifugal and centripetal; positive and negative: interior and exterior. He is a living, breathing, powerful magnet. There is a magnet lying in the midst of splinters of steel. What is the action going on? It attracts, it repels. So also with man. He draws things to himself; he drives things away from himself.

Again, Man acts upon three planes; physical, mental, spiritual. Some are active upon the first only. They are the lowest type of humanity. They are in the thrall of matter. They are in the things of the earth, earthy. They are tied down to the attractions of the world and the flesh. They have their thoughts bound to the physical and carnal side of life. They do not live to eat but eat to live. Their souls say 'eat,' but they cry aloud 'No, you fool, I will feast.' Their souls say 'Man and woman shall be one in the spirit.' But they say, 'No, man and woman shall be one in the flesh.'

One functioning only on a physical plane cossets his body; he kills harmless animals simply to please his palate; his own senses must be constantly gratified by means fair or foul: he it is who says 'Eat, drink and be merry, for tomorrow we die:' 'Ye Gods! I have dined today, tomorrow! do thy worst:' The physical man is the lowest man, the blindworm of fate, the slave of his desire-nature. He is the domestic tyrant; the cruel Shylock insisting upon his pound of flesh; the oppressive ruler; the coarse-fibred, beef-and-beer-bred eater of burnt flesh. The physical man cares little for God except when the wolf is growling at the door. But when pain batters his brow; when his child, whom alone he perhaps loves, is writhing in pain, he thinks of God, goes to church, and prays for the pardon of sins he will commit again, and again and again. How woeful is this state of mind! Yet it is not necessary. We have all been through this experience. So if we come across one such, we must not shun him, but rather we should try our best to give him a lift. He is the object of our compassion and not of hatred. Remember always: Those who hate others for being evil are themselves evil. The face of another man is the mirror in which I dress my own. If I am evil, I shall see others as such. To the jaundiced eye everything appears yellow. My eyes axe blinded by my own evil tendencies. Perhaps I am beginning to fight evil in myself. Hence when I see another worse than myself, I see evil in a magnified form. I therefore feel my indignation rise up against it and I hate the evil man, for is he not the embodiment of what he appears to be? This repulsion is in me because I myself am struggling with evil. The man who is subject to fits of righteous indignation is really himself very imperfect. He instinctively clings to stern rejection of an evil as the only way to escape it. But when your conquest has risen to a height of assurance, you do not hate; you pity; you help.

Now man not being by any means a finished product of Nature, but only a developing creature, full of immense potentialities, cannot, even if he would, remain a permanent fixture in the narrow sphere of the physical senses. Impacts from without, the slings and arrows of adversity, the ups and downs of life, are dashing up against his sleeping consciousness; they are so many blows to open up his mental horizon. It is sufferings that drive lessons home and propel the dormant consciousness along the endless track of spiritual evolution.

Extremes meet. What is the state of the Zoophite or of the stone. Complete absence of thought. Perhaps a faint, imperceptible vibration. Now, tell me what is the state of the highest man—the adept—in the superconscious stage, in Nirvana;—complete suspension of thought, complete quietude of the otherwise intensely active life-forces. Then is the adept in Samadhi the same as the Zoophite? No! No! No! The difference is wide as the ocean. The first is one of intense bliss, the last is one of total inertia.

From this view-point, we can continue the parallel. Man's physical equipment is played upon by three special forces: *Sathva*, *Rajas*, and *Tamas*; rhythm: mobility: inertia. Taking the last first we see that *tamas* is inertia. The *tamasic* man is lazy, dull, inactive, weighed down by his own sensual thoughts. He has no control over himself. He is lifeless. Digestion and sex absorb his vital forces. His formulae of life are Eating, Drinking and Breeding. Having no strength, no inner force of character, resistance of evil is an utter impossibility to him. He plays today to the rich for the loaves and fishes of office. He higgles. He cringes. He weeps. He whines. He goes about trying to please everybody and thus he pleases nobody. The smile of the rich is his sunshine. The empty praise of fools is his crowning victory. When evil presses him down, he cries aloud: "What can I do? I am so weak, such a sinner!" He is thus condemning himself. Unable to resist evil,—for he does not resist but simply sits down and wrings his hands and beats his breast—he hates himself. It is all kismet, is his wail! Ah! this superstition! How vice-like is its grip on the *tamasic* man!

Once upon a time there lived a Persian king who commanded the angelic as well as the human worlds. *Peris*, and *houries* of transcendent charm, slaves, dzins, gods, animals, all obeyed him. This powerful monarch had a very wise physician at his court. This physician was master of all occult knowledge. Vast was his learning—deep his erudition. The finer forces of this tremendous universe had no secrets for him. The king in one of his odd moments sent for him. "Great Master of the Mysterious in Nature, solve me the riddle of birth and death. Solve me the riddle of fate,"—thus spoke the monarch. "Gracious king," replied the physician, "Fate wears an inscrutable face. It sways all, all." "Prove it," challenged the king. The physician then had a jar brought up to him. He prepared certain combinations of herbs, known only to the ancient Kabalists and put them into the jar. He then had the jar hermetically sealed; and handed it to the king: "King! I have gratified your whim. My life's span covers twenty-four hours more. Six months after you shall open this jar in the presence of all your courtiers. Out of the jar shall emerge a bird of royal plumage. Let the bravest man be ready to ride after this bird. Let his steed be of the fleetest and the best in your stud. This bird shall fly over 600 miles. The horseman must follow it alone. It will at last perch itself on a tree of great height. It will then begin to pluck its splendid feathers one by one and eat them up. It will next begin to tear up its legs and eat them up. It will then plunge its beak into its own stomach, and drawing forth the entrails, eat them up, too. Let the horseman stand beneath the tree and watch the bird closely. As soon as the bird has eaten up its whole body except the neck and the head, let him ask it 3 questions and the answers shall be quite correct." Twenty-four hours later this great occultist breathed his last. The king had everything arranged and the physician's son, a young warrior of great prowess, consented to follow the bird. Six months after the jar was opened before the whole court. Up flew a bird of wondrous beauty. Light flashed from its body. With an ear-piercing cry, the bird winged its way through space, the youth riding after him. At last the bird alighted on a tall, stately palm tree and began to eat itself up voraciously. "Now the moment approaches," said the brave youth exultingly. But hardly had he uttered these words than a terrible, acute, unbearable, pain shot through his brain. It was toothache. Whilst the youth was thus writhing in exquisite suffering the bird spoke, "Brave warrior! Be quick. My head and neck remain. Quick! Put the questions or I eat up my neck also." But the youth was crawling in pain. His senses had fled. Yet making an effort he asked, "What is the remedy for toothache?" "Zambur" (the instrument for extracting teeth)— came the ringing reply. "What is the remedy for toothache?" "Zambur," cried the bird again. "What is the remedy for toothache?" "Zambur," sang out the bird for the third time and vanished from sight. The king when he heard it felt deeply chagrined. But what could he say to the youth. "I would have done the same thing!" exclaimed the just monarch sadly, "Who can triumph over fate?"

Therefore conquer the flesh before you question the mysteries of Life. It would be the turning-point in the life of the *tamasic* man if he could say "I will resist evil." His non-resistance is due to weakness and weakness alone. Then comes the *Rajasic* man: full of activity: his brain toned up to a tremendous pitch of energy. "Nothing shall stand in my way," is his determined cry. "I will resist." He does not sit down and bemoan his lot. He does not talk of destiny, his evil star, his guardian angel, his fate. He measures his strength by his resistance of all that would bar his progress. He strikes. He resists evil and thereby does the right thing. He passes through much storm and stress, toil and turmoil, but his spirit burns with a steady blaze. Nothing can crush him. At last this severe and continued fighting so toughens and tones his fibres that he has but to lift a finger in order to bring others to his feet. Then comes calmness. He is a lamp burning steadily despite the winds and waves playing around him. At last, he is conscious of tremendous force. He knows he can smite a fellow down easily. Then possessed of this superhuman strength the saint forbears. He has the power, but wields it for good purposes alone. This is the *Sathvic* man. This is then the supreme stage: *Non-resistance of evil*.

To resume the thread of our discourse: The physical man would gladly remain in the quagmire, but things go against his wishes. His consciousness is trying to individualize itself, to centre itself; and the result of his effort is that he is being flung about mentally. The mind wanders. It is being tossed about. It is the butter-fly mind. The first stage of consciousness. It is called the *kshipta* state.

The next stage is brought about by the breaking of the emotions, the passions, the lust of the flesh, the lust of life, the pride of the eye. When these assert themselves, confusion, utter and most desolate follows. A still small voice is constantly telling, "It is bad to lose your temper," but you never try to keep it till you have lost it. The same with other foibles. You wish to control but you cannot just when you ought to. There comes a feeling of utter ignorance, despair and desolation. Life seems insipid. Pleasures have lost their piquant flavour. You are sad-eyed, silent, yet patiently suffering. The crucifixion nails are being driven in. The pain is acute. This is the *mudha* state. In this transition stage, the individualized consciousness is suffering its birth-pangs. It has yet to cut its wisdom-teeth. The gold is being put into a furnace of fire that the dross may be burnt off and the pure metal come out in all its shining splendor.

But consciousness is a series of sudden awakenings, with a sure belief in its actual existence. Thus at last the man who has been willing earnestly to achieve self-control draws help to himself: Men superior to him mentally and spiritually; books rich with useful information; thoughts laden with force;—all are drawn to him. He hears the great men; receives their higher vibrations; absorbs same. He extracts useful details from books. He pauses in the rush of life when a good thought shines out to him. He is building up an idea] for himself. His life is taking on a coherent shape. He is no more aimless. He has a wider outlook on life. Blissful visions of the perfect man that he is to be one day float before his eyes. Peace comes and folds its wings around his once pain-stricken life for a few moments. No achievement has yet come to him. He is simply surrounded with delicious daydreams. He is thus vitalizing his ideal. At last the ideal possesses him, entrances him, fascinates him. His is in a state of infatuation. He is mad upon one idea. He is turned inwards. Externality is no more his bane. Thus perhaps he goes through life dominated by one idea. This is the third stage: *Vikshipta:* the state of preoccupation through love, ambition, etc. "Genius is madness," they say. So it is. This man is approaching Yoga. He is under the magic spell of a fixed idea. He may under its influence reel off into monomania or he may suffer martyrdom. Maniac or martyr, he stands for an idea. This man, who instead of being possessed by one single idea, possesses it and controls it, touches the higher consciousness.

In the third stage this Eternal Traveller learns *Viveka:* "discrimination between the real and the unreal, between the outer and the inner." In the fourth, he learns *Ekagrata:*—one-pointedness. He carved out a statuesque ideal of himself. He has to actualise it, to vitalise it, to realise it. Now comes the state of practice, of training, of discipline, of asceticism, of austerities, of *vairagya*—dispassion,—of solitude, of utter devotion to his ideal. He is unattached. The world is no longer for him. His whole mind is concentrated, focused, upon his ideal. He is a Stoic of stoics. He is above pleasure and pain, praise and blame, virtue and vice, and all the other dualities. He knows that he cannot have the one without the other. No longer does he tremble. "THERE CAN BE NO FALL NOW," he says. "I live in the ETERNAL. I can never die. My ideal is mine already mentally. I shall bring it down to the physical through continued exertion. I have started the fine causes, I have introduced the thin end of the wedge and each stroke shall drive it deeper." This stage is the fifth stage: *Nirudha:* self-controlled: takes or does not take, chooses as he wills according to the illumined will. This man can effectively practice Yoga. This stage corresponds to activity on the spiritual plane. Further Patanjali tells in that "*these stages of mind are on every plane.*"

Now, my reader, if you are undergoing training, think well over what I have said. It is but little at the best. Yet, it will help teach you to realize your own state. In the first and second stages, Yoga is impossible. In these, you are in the womb of pain. But take heart, thou brave one! Pain is to be accepted. It will chasten, toughen and strengthen you. Hence flinch not.

If in the third, you are nearly ready for the treading of the higher path. Short indeed is the transition from the third to the fourth, from thence to the fifth, and thence to Samadhi. The last you need hardly aim at; so difficult indeed is its achievement that the mere contemplation of it will dash your spirits. Effort, intensity of the will-to-achieve, earnestness, purity, devotion, tenacity of purpose, will bridge the distance of time for you. The light shining upon us is but a fitful glimmer. We shall strengthen it so that it shall burn steadily, calmly, evenly, right on through life. Do you hear this call? It is not a call to arms: to bloodshed: to manslaughter: to worldism: to sham supernaturalism: to present-day spiritualism. It is a call to asceticism;—stern, self-imposed, and severe: to self-sacrifice; to chastity; to manhood; to continence; to mercy; to brotherhood; to life; keener, harder, fuller, more sensitive; to Love, pure and simple. Here you touch the apex of bliss. Here you drink God's sweet, soothing elixir at the pure fount of life. Here you realise all that you have been hungering for. Here learn to say with the dear blessed Swami:

> "Each soul is potentially divine. The Goal is to manifest this divinity within, by controlling nature, external and internal. Do this either by work, or worship, or psychic control, or philosophy, by one or more, or all of these—and be free. This is the whole of religion. Doctrines or dogmas, or rituals, or books, or temples, or forms are but secondary details. "
>
> —*Vivekananda.*

Learn to say these blessed, saving words with your heart full of Divine passion. Learn to rest upon them as you would on a rock. They were ground out of the heart's blood of one of India's greatest saints. Meditate upon them. Make them the flesh of your flesh and the bone of your bone. Rest under the protecting wings for ever and ever. You are great. Compared to your nature this world is but a pinch of star-dust. Lightning can but smite your body at worst, not you. The sword can but cut up your body into pieces, not you. The fire can but burn your body, not you. The water can but drown your body, not you. Why fear then? O Thou Soul! You are Master, not somewhere and sometimes. but everywhere and always. YOU ARE OF GOD.

CONSTRUCTIVE IDEALISM

WHAT is Constructive Idealism?

It is a process whereby we strive to construct, develop and project an ideal personality on the spiritual, mental and physical rungs of human evolution. It is training, self-imposed and self-directed. Man's immediate developmental conditions are, beyond all doubt, thought-structures materialised on the physical plane, since Man is ever the reflex of his mind. Could we lift the brain-cap of a man and watch the inter-play of Will, Emotion and Intellect, we should in no time become convinced that our thought-life has never lost the grand and stern emphasis of its dignity. But it is given to us to make or mar, to raise or to lower ourselves.

Efforts to call up the resurgence of the spiritual forces that inhere in us and that are interaffinitised to the psychic realms of vibration are so many blood-drops from the core of our being sprinkled upon fertile soil. Our reaction upon Nature determines the centre and turning-point of our life. This reaction is due to the action of the Free-Will. The Will is the pivotal point round which revolve the issues of destiny. Constructive Idealism then is a life-building assimilation of the highest and the best within the reach of our mental and spiritual vision. It is from my point of view a determined effort to intensify ourselves along lines of human uplift by a systematized application of the laws of psychology. It is the putting forth of positive effort to develop and expand our spiritual stature. Life in this world is a gymnasium for the exercise of the will. It matters little how many years you h been here in this world. It matters little how many moments of sense enjoyment you have had. Indeed! You may be as old as Methuselah., Your entire life-span may have been enjoyable. Such things do not count. What is of vital moment is how far you have succeeded in your triumph over your lower Nature, how far your Spirituality, Firmness, Conscientiousness, Veneration, Causality, etc., are developed; how far you feel for suffering humanity; how far your Soul is on the ascendant and your flesh is under your feet. For this last is the crown and climax of all human endeavor along right lines. It is chastity alone that can give us a lift up from the quadruped stage. With ordinary humanity, with even the intellectual classes—in some measure—it is a step forward and then a long stagger backwards to the animal stage. This phenomenon is so constant that the aspiring soul stops, hesitates, and then as if a douche of cold water had been poured upon it, shrivels up in fear and heaves a sigh, "Oh! It is impossible! It is my nature! How can I transcend it? Impossible! Impossible!" Poor Ignorant Man! How he weeps and wails. He does not know that nothing is impossible to the Divine Spirit; that there is ever a way out; that there is ever a way up, if its vision were a bit wider and better trained. Know, My Reader! What is soul-force inside of yourself is the mighty Law of God outside; and relief and joy are dependent upon pre-established harmony between the two, for at the center they are One.

Is it possible then? What? Self-conquest? Yes. You can conquer, even utterly crush the lower nature. If it be within range of practicability, why then is the major portion of humanity grovelling in carnality. Because, they do so willingly. It is the animal soul that has fastened its grip upon them. The Higher Soul has been almost buried under coating after coating of carnal tendencies. Man has not obeyed his inmost thought. He has ever yielded to his impulses. He has had his face in a bush and ostrich-like he has considered himself safe. The memories of superstition; the blotted pictures of Heaven and Hell; the preacher of religious dogmas; know-nothing religions, slave-trading and slave-trading religions; the squalor of animal lust, greed, and hard selfism, and every other stripe of absurdity that stalks the land often under the cloak of religion, have so magnetized the eyes of man that he sees nothing better, higher and purer.

Today, materialism has lost not a bit of the old emphasis of its personality, although people struggle hard to dress it up in a clean shirt and present it to the world at large under the guise of religion. Today, more than ever, is the grim hand of the butcher clotted with gore and shambles reek with the blood of innocent animals. The cry transpierces the heavens, yet the ears of man are hermetically sealed. Today, more than ever, does a pious demeanor cover scarlet indulgence. Indeed! Man is lifting the veil from dark proceedings and striving to justify them to our eyes. Hence, more misery, more pain.

Is it possible then to go beyond the lower Nature? Not to flatter the intellect by feeding it upon dirty and unclean garbage, but to expand it to the light of Reason; not to pass the lazy hour but to press it into substantial service; not to pander to the flesh but to render it a clean and fitting temple for the sojourn of the spirit; not to flinch from pain in creep-mouse style, but to face it resolutely, if need be, and make it yield up its last lesson; not to move along lines of least resistance but to set the will against all else; not to wish for and accept ease but to live and breathe for the joy of others:—this line of plain-living and high thinking is a decided step out of a chalk circle of imbecility into strong doing.

You have to develop a life-purpose. Our work is our life-preserver. Remember: "Life only avails, not the having lived. Power ceases in the instant of repose: it resides in the moment of transition from a past state into a new state, in the shooting of the gulf, in the darting to an aim." You must reach out to the highest and the best within the sphere of your vision. Thus alone can you stand out of the deep rut formed by ages of crass ignorance. Your ideal must compel your entire being. There must be tugging hard at the center of your being and earnest longing to live up to the highest within you.

Perhaps it is the flesh that reacts so viciously upon your efforts, your doings and thinkings. Perhaps it is a hypersensitive nervous system that has dragged you on to a low plane of living. Perhaps it is a weak mind that would neither be coaxed out, nor dragged out, nor be lashed out of its chronic condition of fearfulness, general depression, sluggishness, despair and melancholy, worry, hurry and flurry, jealousy, fretfulness, and all-consuming hatred, that sees obstacles where there are none; that is so delicately hinged that a slight feather's weight tips the beam; or a breath of air flings wide the doors to perdition and you are sent flying into the Slough of Despond. Perhaps anxious thoughts loom large, threaten and then destroy repose.

What a catalogue of weaknesses in human nature! Yet, is it not all fact? Morbid thoughts, impure desires, self-pity, painful introspection, continual anticipation of perpetual loss, constant dwelling on a lazy ideal, pessimism, causeless apprehensions,—all these and many more are the pitiless enemies and life long associates of a negative, resistless, nerveless, will-less cast of mind;—a mind void of stamina,—a character out of joint with the laws of right-living and right-thinking. Heredity, environmental conditions, emotion, and ignorance;—all contribute their quota to the emasculation of man's resistant forces. Fact is, men are as lazy as they dare to be. If they work at all, there must be a strong incentive to back up their sudden fit of activity. It is the prospect of an ease-living, lazy life that allures them to activity. It is a long spell of active inactivity that most people want. No wonder their powers of resistance are in a state of atrophy! No wonder they land themselves in a vicious circle! Truly, most truly, has it been said that an idle brain is the devil's workshop. Now, reader, are you one such? I hope not. But, if so, why so? Listen to one of Maeterlinck's symbolic stories.

In the middle ages there lived a powerful man who was impressed by the fact that each wish that he had conceived had caused him years of toil, struggle, and hard exertion before it could be accomplished and that, too, when he was on the verge of failure. He could not understand why success was so hard to achieve. He thought hard and searched much. At last he felt that there was a secret enemy that constantly antagonised him. He determined to find him out and crush him. The rugged side of life repelled him. He wished to press on to the fascinating by-ways of pleasure and ease. Life under old conditions was not worth living. This barrier removed, he could be happy. One evening while out walking he saw a man approaching him and he "intuitively, identified" him as his evil genius. He resolved to destroy him. When he came closer, his enemy was discovered as being masked so that none could see his features. "You are the man," said he, in resolute tones, "who from my youth has been thwarting my purposes and nearly defeating me. I am resolved to kill you, and yet am constrained to give you a single chance for life. Draw and defend yourself." "I am at your service," replied the stranger, as he drew his sword, "but before we fight, I want you to identify me." Upon which he drew off his mask and the challenger found that he stood before himself: "Thought." So it is with all of us. Do you remember that song of Omar Khayyam's:

> I sent my soul into the Invisible,
> Some message of the after-life to spell,
> And by-and-by my soul returned to me,
> And answered 'I myself am heav'n and hell.'

There you are! Nothing could be more pointed. We men and women carry our own racks and stretch ourselves thereupon as often as we dash up against the immutable laws of God. Whose aid would you invoke? The question that I would put to you is: Are you victimisable? Are you willingly so? Are you waiting for things to drop from the skies? Ten to one, you are. Then there is no way out, indeed! The first requisite in Constructive Idealism is self-reliance. You simply must kick away all props. You must stand upon your own feet. Thus poised you are at the top of your condition. Once you have nerved yourself to fight your battles on your own private strength, I see no limits to your ascending force. This determination will arm you with weapons none can conquer. All depends upon the strength, intensity and elasticity of your resolution to act from your own centre. All power resides in you. This is the first, last and the only lesson the student of Occultism has to master. Locked up in your soul is to be found Infinite Knowledge, Infinite Existence, Infinite Bliss. The more you learn to tap your soul-forces with confidence the surer your power over yourself and hence over others.

Each soul, individually, exists on earth to fulfil a mission which it alone can fulfil. Most wisely does Dr. Sanjivi say "Your existence is no accident but is a representative of Life and what Life is." Quite so. You are here because you are (indeed!) a necessity, an indispensable something which nature requires for the execution of certain designs. No more of foreign supports then. You have to stand alone; thus alone will strength flow into your veins. All power is inborn. It is never an accretion from without. Those that go careering madly into the external world are like men standing upon their heads instead of on their feet. Those that turn ever inwards for inspiration, for strength, stand aright, command their limbs, and work miracles. They are as firm columns sustaining immense fabrics. Yes, cat-like you must ever fall upon your feet. Trust yourself and in the endless mutation of things you shall discover that naught can establish you in peace but yourself. Do you remember Napoleon's masterly advice to his elder brother Joseph? It was compressed in two words: "Be Master." Sturdy natures are not leaning willows. They act from within, from themselves. It is these that shed healing by their mere presence. It is these that have tossed overboard idolatries, customs and conventions. They do not seek for compassion. Indeed they resent all gratis sympathy. With self-trust new powers are born. For everything at the core is wrought out of one hidden stuff. We read in our scriptures how Uddalaka taught his son this truth by salt dissolved in water. The boy was required to take a solution of salt and water. Next day the father asked him for the salt. The boy could not find it. "Taste from the top," said the father. "It is saltish," replied the boy. "Taste from the middle of the water." "It is saltish," replied the boy. "Taste from the bottom," enjoined the father. "It is saltish." Now, so it is with the Universal Soul—the Over-Soul. It is the One, the indivisible Spirit running through entire nature, vivifying all, sustaining all, evolving in all. It is this bridge that spans the "gulf" that Tyndall said could never be bridged over.

The salt disappeared but it pervaded the entire water. Then Uddalaka said, "It is the Universal Self, O Svethaketu! Thou art That." True.

The naturalist is right in his tracing of the same type under every metamorphosis. A horse is a running man. A fish is a swimming man. A bird is a flying man. A tree is a rooted man. So says Emerson. Further, to believe your own thought, to believe that what is true for you in your private heart is true for all men—that is genius. Is it not high time then that you resolved to take yourself for better, for worse? In rejecting yourself, in wishing that you were Mr. or Mrs. So-and-So instead of what you are, in imitating others, in bemoaning your lot, you are denying God in the only form He can ever express in Man—Faith—Faith-in-your-self. Said Vivekananda, 'Have that tremendous faith in yourself which I had when I was a child and I have been working it out in my life! I have quoted from memory. Yet I well remember those words, "Tremendous faith in yourself" Listen again, "There is a time in every man's education when he arrives at the conviction that envy is ignorance; that imitation is suicide;—that though the whole universe is full of good, no kernel of nourishing corn can come to him but through his toil bestowed on that piece of ground which is given to him to till." We know ourselves only when we have tried to do so and not before. Therefore say, "Henceforth things must take a new scale from me. I obey no law but what is sanctioned by my own judgment. I am a disembodied spirit working, living and breathing for whatever is related to me by spiritual affinity. I care little for this world with its thousand-cloven tongues of gratis advice, praise and censure. I can but obey my polarity. I want nothing. I seek strength in chastity. I seek wisdom in the silence of my own heart. Death shall wring from me but one pang and not even that if I can help it. I shall be calm. Naught shall ruffle my calm. For each time I feel the stabs of anxiety and remorse I die. The Lord is my refuge. I can only live under His control." This is the doctrine of fearlessness. For says Zoroaster: "To the persevering mortal the blessed immortals are swift." Some men think they can well afford to be lazy, since everyone is working and so far as 1 am concerned I do not see why all life should be labor. This is a serious self-deception indeed! Our share of work is to persevere in the path of absolute purity.

Once upon a time there was a king who had a very large number of courtiers. Now courtiers are flatterers, born deceivers. They all swore to the king that each one of them was ready to sacrifice his life for the king. The king was mightily pleased. At this time there appeared a Sanyasin from some place at the King's Court. The king, like all vain people, told the

Sanyasin that there never before had been a king for whom his entire number of courtiers was ready to sacrifice their lives. The Sanyasin smiled incredulously and told our king that he did not believe it. "Put them to the test," said the king. The Sanyasin then had it proclaimed that he was going to hold a sacrifice whereby great advantages would accrue to the king. His only condition was that each courtier should go alone to a tank and pour a pitcher of milk thereinto in the dark of night. "Is that all?" asked the king in surprise. "Yes," replied the Sanyasin. Next morning the king visited the tank which instead of being full of milk was full of water. Each one of the courtiers had thought he could afford to practice deception and poured in a pitcherful of water.

So also the present generation of India. 'Oh! There are great Yogis in the forest making tapas for the good of the world. I need not trouble. I can well be spared.' No! No! You cannot be spared. There is not one soul that can snap asunder the bond of Divine Brotherhood. If you, who are young and vigorous, are abusing your advantages by letting them slip by through your lazy and selfish propensities, then know that a time will come when you will look for them in vain. *If you will not when you may, you shall not when you will.* I see young men who have all possible chances allowed them. Nothing weighs upon their minds. Yet these complain loudest. Poor Souls! Instead of working now while the sun shines upon them, they are content to lead aimless lives. Man's work is his inner development and unfoldment. Those who are fully alive to this fact can never be satisfied with living at low pressure. It is the pitch at which a man lives that counts most. Everything concentrates. Diffusion leads to confusion. "Not they that eat most, but they that digest most are the most nourished. Not they that get most but they that keep and give the most, are the richest. So not they that hear most, or read most, but they that meditate most and pray most and in the silent mystic way of Love give out the most are the most edified and nourished and enriched unto everlasting life, here, now, and forever. "Meditate upon these things," and "As thy days pass so shall thy strength be." Therefore, shut yourself up in your room and with strenuous and earnest zeal, go on adding stroke after stroke of steady work for your soul-expression. Results will come in their own good time and that moment is best for you and the world when you get great gleams of light from your higher nature.

HIGHER REASON AND JUDGMENT

ANOTHER requisite is Fearlessness. "What a tiresome rigmarole of requisites! I know it all!" you may say. But you don't! I, too, thought so years ago. You have to take them up and meditate upon them. Thus alone can they become inwoven with your nature. Few people possess this virtue. It has to be cultivated with assiduous zeal before you can proceed a step further. Now just turn in and examine yourself in the calm light of reason. See! You have given your body first place right along. You have grown quite fond of it. Your life consists in taking care of and yielding to the demands of your physical nature. No wonder then that you are still the slave of carnal tendencies. A force far mightier than yourself seems to grip you, overbear your feeble will and whirl you where it will. Resolve this moment to be chaste and continent in thought, word and deed, and ten to one but that you will be faced by a veritable host of evil forces forming around you a ring-pass-not from which you cannot effect an escape; struggle, foam, fume and wrestle as you will. You fall into quick-sands which you would but cannot avoid. You have ever moved along lines of least resistance. You fancied yourself in fine condition indeed! You laughed your vacuous, unmanly, ignorant laugh against those who are ever serious, austere, and plodding. You considered these as sorely ridden hacks who have naught of the pleasures of life to engage them. Though you quailed abjectly beneath their sad, stern glance, you shot witty things against them when their backs were turned. You had even the impudence to admonish them against austere and abstemious ways.

Now the scales have dropped from your eyes: you who sat in the seat of the scornful and passed judgment on others; How you wish somebody would come to your rescue and lift you bodily out of this Pit of Trophet! But mere lifting won't do at all. You will drift back again. You have to be born again. A spiritual regeneration is called for. Serious introspection must be a constant virtue. Why do you fear? Because you are afraid of Fear, your relentless Hierophant. That is the causeless cause of fear. Secondly because you are so fond of your skin. Thirdly because Nature won't let you off. Time was when you lived, breathed and enjoyed evil. Your disgraceful past is reacting with all the cumulative force of evil-doing and what is far more heinous, evil thinking. You have been running in accustomed grooves. Now is the time to turn over a new leaf. Your salvation lies in these: 1. First and foremost, resolve not to give way to Fear, for there is Nothing to fear but Fear. Philosophy will come to your help, as I hope to show you later on. 2. Then you must renounce your love for the flesh. It is a hard task. But I can see no other way out. I shall tell you the 'how' of it. It rests with you to accept or refuse. 3. Learn to be patient under suffering. Your Karma must work itself out. But you can neutralise its force in proportion to your earnestness in following my advice to the letter. Now for the remedial aspect of philosophy.

The aim of philosophy is to put an end to pain. Your fear has, back of it, a shrinking from pain. Is pain then so unwelcome? Edward Carpenter in his beautiful poem "Man and Satan" says "Every pain that I suffered in one body became a power which I wielded in the next." The functions of pain are fivefold. The nature of the Atman—the individualised self incarnation—is all-blissfulness. Time is an excrescence. It is Not-self. The law of evolution is Manifestation. There are two paths. The one is *Pravritti*. It signifies "revolving towards." The other is "*Nivritti*: revolving away." The vast mass of humanity are treading the former. The powers of the soul must be turned outwards, focused upon the external world, in order that it may acquire a knowledge of it. The soul is embosomed in rapture. It is ever inward-turned. In order that it may wake up from its latent condition and find expression physically, it must be impinged upon by pain. If there be a continued influx of streams of bliss, no power would manifest. When water is allowed its free course, it flows on smoothly. But just put a bar across its onflow. How it struggles, hisses and fumes in order to get rid of the barrier! Now you understand why the will arms itself with sudden force when the lash of disgrace and contumely stirs it up. The greater the stirring and the more continued the spasm of pain, the deeper the impression left upon the memory, the fiercer the out-put of soul energy. When it is a gentle twinge only, the soul turns over like the proverbial sleepy boy and forgets it instantly. You repeat your folly. Now our psychology fixes itself ever on the ultimate analysis of fact. Hence Vyasa in his commentary on Patanjali gives pain the first seat as an important factor that goes to build up the Causal Body—the *Karana Sharira*, or the receptacle in which lie all the seeds of actions—the proper development of which blazes the way to Self-realisation.

The first and most important function of pain is to call out the activity-aspect of the soul. Remember it has no permanent place. Take your cue and learn to love exertion, and pain shall not come. The next function of pain is to establish rhythmic conditions in the physical form. It organises the body aright. I have told you in my paper on "Man's Divine Heritage" how the transition to peace must always be through struggle and painful fighting. Says the Lord Sri Krishna in the Bhagavad Gita:—1. That is like poison at first, but nectar at the end, that happiness is declared Satvic, born of the translucence of the intellect due to Self-realisation. 2. That which arises from the contact of object with sense, at first like nectar, but at the end like poison, that happiness is declared to be Rajasic. 3. That happiness which begins and ends in self-delusion arising from sleep, indolence and miscomprehension, that is declared to be Tamasic. 4. There is no entity on earth, or again in heaven among the Devas that is devoid of these three Gunas, born of Prakriti. 5. Control of mind and senses, austerity, purity, forbearance, and also uprightness, knowledge, realisation, belief in the hereafter—these are the ways of the Satvic.

Thus you see that the putting forth of positive effort, spoken of already, will go to effectively shake out the grosser and coarsened forms of vibrations in the body. Exertion will organise your brain, develop and unfold its powers. The grind of intellectual training means pain in its exquisite form for the tamasic man. Austere living is just what man hates. Sense-pleasures he eagerly seeks. Just as exercise in the physical sense is painful to begin with, so it causes more life to flow into your muscles, nerves and fibres; and development results. Nothing has seemed to you more painful than the deliberate development of the Will. It is most painful at first. Yet, if you have done it or if you ever do it, you shall know that the harmonic poise of the Will-power is the mightiest aspect of Power in man. Well, then, this is the third function of pain. It develops power. "Power is pain transmuted."

Read the life of Napoleon. There you see the finest manifestation of power. This man small and insignificant of build commanded the rugged soldiers as if they were infants. They were as wax in his hands. He could mould them as he wished. Take this single instance. Napoleon hearing that the Bourbons were misgoverning his country, returned from his exile at Elba. He had to give the guards the slip. He returned with no forces. He was alone in the midst of his bitterest enemies, the Bourbons. Troops were drawn up to fight him. The entire army had been commanded to fire at his breast. They were standing—the Bourbon soldiers—with their muskets levelled at his breast ready for the command "Aim." Napoleon on foot, alone, undefended and unarmed, marched deliberately towards the troops with measured tread, gazing directly into their eyes. The command to "Fire" was shouted out. A single shot would have killed him. A fortune would have awaited the man who fired it. If the army had obeyed the order no less than forty thousand bullets would have entered Napoleon's breast. But this man flinched not. He undid the buttons, bared his breast and stood within a few yards facing them. The whole army wavered. How could they shoot this man? "Fire!" "Fire!!" But how could they fire? They were under this man's fascination. They were spell-bound. They couldn't fire. Not one man obeyed the order. Not one, mark you, out of these thousands! They all threw down their guns and ran to him, shouting "Vive l'Empereur!" Yet if you turn to this man's early life, you see him imposing the most painful tasks upon himself. For days he would go without sleep, rest and food, deeply absorbed in study. His hard labours at his studies in early life dwarfed his stature. His appearance at times, we read, was woeful to contemplate because of his painful hardships. But then there was lightning in his eyes which burned and flashed with the fire of his spirit. Truly, most truly, is "pain" transmuted into "Power."

The Yogi whose severe austerities strike you dumb with surprise and horror, tames the lions and tigers of the forest simply by a look. In point of fact all advanced Yogis have this and thousands of other such wonderful powers. The fourth function is that pain purifies. "Slowly and resolutely as a fly cleans its legs of the honey in which it has been caught—so remove thou, if it be only for a time, every particle which sullies the brightness of thy mind. Return into thyself content to give but asking no one—asking nothing."

Now this cleansing process you set about only under the crucifixion of pain. Human nature is obdurate. For ages the animal propensities have been developed. Unless drastic methods be employed they are impossible of subjugation. There is nothing like pain as a teacher. Because first it is a purifier. Once your nature has been passed through the fire of suffering it will have known the serious side of life. It will represent sterner stuff than the mere gibbering, imitative tendencies of the ape.

Next pain is a discipliner of mind and body. Now if you remember all this, you will be patient under suffering. You will not tug and pull, gnash your teeth and break down. You will be indifferent alike to pain and pleasure. For as you study and meditate, as wisdom opens out to your vision, you shall see that there is ever a cause behind. You shall go on calmly working for higher ends, not waiting for release as a condition of work.

Then there are other reasons why you should not give way to fear. Says Professor James "There is no sort of consciousness whatever, be it sensation, feeling or idea, which does not directly and of itself discharge into some motor effect." Says Tichner "It is a rule without exception that every mental process has in its condition a bodily process, some change in the central nervous system and more particularly in the cerebral cortex. No psychosis without neurosis. There is no mental state which has not a peculiar nervous state corresponding to it." A Mental Healer of wide influence says "Just as truly as faith is a talisman by which we can successfully conjure, so is fear a palsy by which disaster is insured." Rev. Tarley T. Womer tells us the following story: It is said that a certain man tried to kill his wife by throwing her from a boat while they were crossing a river. The woman kept herself from sinking by holding on to the side of the boat. In his furious rage the man struck her with an axe and severed two of her fingers. But somehow she was rescued and later on a reconciliation was effected and they lived together happily. But for several succeeding generations every male child that was born to the family had two fingers missing.

Your thoughts effect your body just as they shape your destiny. Fear thoughts, worrisome and melancholy thoughts destroy brain cells and smash down the tissue walls, take the light out of your eyes, poison your blood, lower your vitality and write O Coward! Coward!! on your forehead. Whereas the positive will is a strong shield from which all destructive forces glance off like so many wisps of straw. So long as we cling to this body, we give the spirit but small chance of asserting itself. Our thoughts are bound to the physical and carnal side of life. Our eyes have the mud of materialism in them. But just register a vow that you will ever contemplate and stand by the Spirit, and try ever to realise it and the heavens will clear out for you. Life, though serious and stern, shall reflect power; shall shed healing and flash with the light of the Spirit. If not, why not? Because, sir, you are still not earnest, still animalised. I say "It is possible. Perfectly possible." I have a right to say it. I have seen it with my own eyes. Others do it. Why can't you? Nature's laws are rigid and uniform in their working. What one man can do others must be able to do. Instead of one man, thousands of the children of India are doing it.

All aspirants after Occultism have to set before themselves as a first step the conquest of the physical nature. The Sanyasin is not permitted to remain under the same roof for more than a day;—at the most three days. He has given up his body. He knows it is the mortal, the grosser side of his nature. He trains it after certain methods; purifies and subdues it, that done, he is free. He is non-attached. He is the master. He can turn the full current of his life-forces upon a single thought, and so vitalise it with the electric principle in himself that it shall have all the potency of the charged wires of a dynamo.

There has gone out a foolish and unpardonable impression from some ignorant Western writers that the Yogi is an air-fed, emaciated, human wreck. Yes! You Westerns would give way under these practices. You who are such staunch believers in nourishment and nutrition could hardly believe the Swami Dharmananda Mahavarati when he says: In the beginning of the year 18.. I formed the acquaintance of a Yogi who was then in his 260th year. In another year on my way from Afghanistan I was highly delighted at seeing a Jain woman (a Yogini) whose age could be ascertained from her eyelashes which grew again but had not turned grey. She was about 500 years old! Barth on yoga exercises says "I conscientiously observed they can only end in folly and idiocy." Professor Huxley calls them delusions! The face of Vivekananda is not a strange one to my American readers. Is that inspiring appearance indicative of mental aberration? Now listen to his account of himself: Many times I have been in the jaws of death, starving, footsore and weary; for days and days I had had no food! and often could walk no farther; I would sink down under a tree and life would seem ebbing away. I could not speak, I could scarcely think, but at last the mind would revert to the idea: "I have no fear of death; I never hunger nor thirst. The whole of nature cannot crush me; it is my servant. Assert thy strength, thou Lord of Lords! Regain thy lost empire! Arise and walk and stop not, and I would rise up, reinvigorated, and here am I, living today. This is our Swamin! Strong as a rock and one of India's Yogis. This man lived in mountain caves for years. He climbed over the mountains on foot to Thibet. He is by no means a solitary instance. Now reader! If you are wise, you will meditate day after day on these things. The practical lessons will follow. In the meantime fear not."

CONQUEST OF FEAR

"There is Nothing to Fear But Fear."

FEAR is one of the cardinal emotions that result from the play of certain forces in the human personality. Our emotional nature is not our Self. I was amused to read in a Phrenological magazine various remarks from certain learned Westerners on the nature and attributes of the Soul. The question was "What is the Soul?" One of the writers insisted upon having this theory accepted by his readers: that the soul has its seat in the organs of Philoprogenitiveness and Friendship. Another one defines these two words as (1) Parental Love and (2) Sociability and Union of Friends. To my readers the fallacy of their statements ought to be quite plain. Our emotions, Love (in the lower phases), Hate, Anger, Fear, etc., bear a direct relation to the external world. When the Intellect dwells upon a desire with a view to externalise or realise the latter, emotion results. It is thus the reaction of the Ego upon sense-impressions received from the objective universe. They have a purely physio-psychological origin and must not be confused with our Soul-processes which are due to the Divine Urge from within, ever impelling the Spirit to express itself upon matter through more and more improved types of personality. Stop right now and understand: Your mission was to energise upon matter, to be master and not slaves. But instead of setting about your business like a master you took hold of the wrong end of the stick and became attached, nay, identified yourself with your forms. This is the supreme tragedy of Maya: Man forgot himself.

What was the result? Ignorance;—and that developed fear. Just view yourself from a physical standpoint. What are you? Are you any more than a geometrical point, a mere human atom in a sea of tremendous forces that could crush you—the form of flesh—in no time. There are monsters—seismic disturbances, cataclysms, earthquakes, famines, gravity, lightning and what not! I need hardly mention the Halley's comet scare to illustrate my point. There is no escaping it that way. Consider yourself as a sack of blood, bone, muscle, cell-stuff and nerve force and you are eternally damned.

No, the remedy lies the other way. That remedy is a sovereign remedy. You must give up your life, if you are to live truly. Sri Krishna taught it in the Gita. He called it Vairagya: Dispassion: Non-attachment: Renunciation. Here is the antidote. Open your Gita and read, "Weapons pierce not the Real Man nor doth the fire burn him; the water affecteth him not; nor the wind drieth him, nor bloweth him away. For he is impregnable and impervious to these things of change—he is eternal, permanent, unchangeable and unalterable—and Real."

You must understand your own nature, if you are to be Fearless. How? You will at once ask me that question. My answer is: Learn to draw inwards and upwards. The lower mind ever darts outwards. This is the sense-born brain that you read of in Western works on Psychology generally. It rests on sensation. It is enthralled by the limitations of temperament, heredity, environment, and the sheaths and clogs of organization. It can only function on the plane of Instinctivity. The way to conquer this mind was pointed out in the Gita when Arjuna complained that it was impetuous, hard to crib as the wind, ever moving outwards, ever restless. The warrior prince was famed for his prowess; had faced strong foes and vanquished them; yet even he cowered before the impetuous rush of this mind; even he broke down in despair. Why not?

Look at the so-called great men of modern times. How full of pride and approach-me-at-your-peril sort of hauteur they are! Just watch them when their "material" or "social" self stands threatened by some approaching danger. Gone is their inflated self-esteem. The whip has not yet been applied; yet they shrink before the terrors of their imagination. Let me say once more, that the worldly man, the purse-proud man, is proud and conceited because his mind is befogged with the fumes of ignorance; a moment shall come when he shall have to face the terrors of his animal soul! then he must fight on his individual strength; he will cry for help from outside but none shall come; the world of the senses which ensnared his mind so long, shall drop away; and the Higher Self must then overcome the Lower. Many are the birth-pangs, but the end,—the goal—justifies the means.

Now turn to Shri Krishna's reply, which alone can solve this riddle for you: Without doubt, O Mighty-armed, the mind is hard to curb and restless but it may be curbed by constant practice (Abhyasa) and dispassion (Vairagya). The student must renounce, once for ever, all that pertains to his Lower

Self and thus pull up the weeds that crowd the soil of his mind. The supreme result of Renunciation is that it enables you to leap from your present position, where there are a thousand strings tugging at your heart; and prepares the way for the inrush of higher, loftier thoughts. By practice is meant constant and unremitting effort at control of the mind, which, by the way, is a science by itself and may be handled later on.

Now, brother, renounce mentally, all attachment to impermanent ends. Dedicate yourself to the Higher Life. The more completely you can do so, the greater the influx of light, the clearer your vision spiritually. You fear because you are laboring under the evil suggestions of your brain-born intellect. As you succeed in "giving up," your soul shall expand and burst asunder 'the clinging chains of the senses,' which breed Fear through Ignorance. Resolve, to be perfectly "Fearless" and so shall you be according to the strength of your resolution.

THE ROLE OF PRAYER

O Lord purify us with water, purify us with solar rays, purify us with medicinal herbs and, above all, purify us with Wisdom, i.e., endow us with POWERS OF MIND by enlightening our intellects.—Rig Veda—viii, 19-2.

HOW exquisitely painful are the effects of Ignorance. Many are the victims, many the bond slaves of their lower selves. Many are the wrecks awaiting an early grave and looking forward to the time when Death shall come as a welcome relief. Many walk the earth with an uneasy Conscience, starting with sudden fright at their own shadows and conscious all the while as if the brand of Cain had burnt its mark on their brows. Many are even now undergoing the tortures of Hell in the fierce conflicts raging in their souls. Many close their eyes when the cold hands of Death have seized upon them with this saddening cry, "To what end have I lived? Alas! I die as ignorant as I was born. All my fond wishes have vanished into thin vapor, all my long cherished aims have been shattered into pieces." Such are the woes of Mankind—God's children.

WHY?

"Ignorance is the only soil where Evils can grow and germinate"—so says Patanjali. The misdirection of Nature's forces entails misery, pain and sorrow. These latter seem quite in advance of the enormity of the mistake. "Why should I be smitten so hard for a little thing like that?" that is the angry protest of the sufferer. I shall take it that you have aspired after noble heights of Spiritual Development and the PEACE consequent thereupon. As Emerson puts it: "Let us say then frankly that the education of the Will is the object of our existence. Poverty, the prison, the rack, the fire, the hatred and execration of our fellow-men appear trials beyond the endurance of common humanity, but to the hero whose intellect is aggrandized by the Soul, and so measures the good which his thought surveys against these penalties; the terrors vanish as darkness at sunrise."

Have you ever caught a glimpse of the peace that passeth all understanding? Let us listen attentively to what a noble thinker says: "There are moments, supreme and rare moments, that come to the life of the pure and the spiritual when every sheath (the material coatings in and through which the spirit impresses its will upon the Objective Universe) is still and harmonious; when the senses are tranquil, quiet, insensitive; when the mind is serene, calm, and unchanging; when, fixed in meditation, the whole being is steady and nothing that is without may avail to disturb; when love has permeated every fibre; when devotion has illuminated, so that the whole nature is translucent; there is a silence and in the silence is a sudden change; no words may tell it; no syllable may utter it, but the change is there; all limitations have fallen away. Every limit of every kind has vanished. As stars swing in boundless space, the self is in limitless life and knows no limits and realizes no bounds. There is light in wisdom, consciousness of perfect light that knows no shadow and therefore knows not itself a slight; the thinker has become the knower; all reason has vanished and all-wisdom has taken its place. Who shall say what it is save that it is bliss? Who shall try to utter that which is unutterable in mortal speech—but it is true and it exists, . . . Its nature is bliss; all the spheres have ceased; all else has gone; none but the pure may reach it; none but the devotee may know it; none but the wise may enter it."

Such indeed is the ineffable sense of power serene that folds its wings around the earnest Yogi. The restless world with its warring interests, its corroding passions, its bloody wars, its existence of want-and-have, of buy-and-sell, of self-love, greed and eternal heart-burn, seems to lose its jar and shock in the presence of this tremendous spiritual force. How can it be otherwise? I take it that your gaze is fixed with earnest longing upon the eternal; that your intellect has expanded to the light of the spiritual illumination, yet,—I cannot help feeling it—so imperfectly, that my aim is, in these short papers, to point out to you the "How" rather than the "Why;" since, from my point of view, the former alone solves the latter; realization alone vanquishes the weapons of skepticism and doubt. "Steadfastly by truth, by austerity, by perfect wisdom, by Brahmacharya-practice (Perfect Chastity) is this atma attained. In the midst of the body, clad in light, He whom the sinless and the subdued behold is pure."—(Mundakopanishad).

Feel convinced, student, that the emotion which impels to lofty aspiration and noble achievement is powerless in itself, unless the clear light of expanded intellect irradiates the soul and shines full along your path. "The intellect," said Sextus the Pythagorean, "is a chorus of Divinities. From the plane of pure intellection all life, both subjective and objective, both inner and outer, appears embosomed in beauty, but, viewed from the platform of action, life is a struggle, where the stakes are life and death, and in which "The joys of conquest are the joys of man." In the supreme struggle for Self Perfection,—for you must aim at nothing short of that,—the joys of the final triumph constitute the greatest joy of man.

Nowadays it is the way with some to run down the intellect and to give emotions the first place. Again, there are others who ask you to kill out the heart—the seat of emotion—and to give the head—the seat of reason—the first place. Both schools are dogmatic and their reasoning is shallow, very shallow. The fact is;—neither can be suppressed and crushed out. Steady reflection will prove that each is great in its own place, that the heart and the head, the feelings and the intelligence, complement themselves, and both are ultimately resolvable into Infinity—which is Unity, pure and simple. Nature aims at human development on all planes and you must unfold on all sides; otherwise you run the great risk of being top-heavy, onesided, fanatical, narrow and short-sighted. Indeed, you cannot infringe upon the Eternal Law of all-round development without bringing pain upon yourself. Try to realize this supreme truth! Nature is conquered by Obedience. Nature's laws are invariable and their very uniformity is your safeguard. Knowledge invests you with the power to control. Nature's forces are at your disposal and you must learn how to manipulate them. If you put the same question to Nature rightly, the same answers shall be invariably returned. When the scientist in the laboratory fails to perfect an experiment, he examines his methods and always finds somewhere something wrong in his own processes.

Hence, if you plead ignorance as the cause of your blunders all blame to you and do not be surprised if dire punishment overtakes you for pulling the strings of fate the wrong way. This is at the root of all human miseries. Now, there are those who pretend to laugh at the efficacy of the intellect to promote spiritual development. They laugh at Yoga and austere living and say, "O, everything comes from devotion and worship. God will give me everything." Quite so. Perfectly so. But friend, how is it that after you have had your tear—relief from your little, emotionally-worded prayer, you seem to forget everything but your personal concerns; you seem thoroughly steeped in animalism, selflove and hatred; you seem quite upset at the loss of your trifling worldly things; you seem swayed to and fro by other's opinions; by your own passions. Come, are you not a slave? Would you dare to part with your fleshy tenement at a moment's notice? Are you not far removed from God?

Then, how dare you cry down the Yogi and his efforts to master himself? I say, how dare you? You profess to follow the dictates of the heart and yet your egg-shell existence of narrow selfism has quite dried up the fountain of love within you. No; so long as you are a slave, you cannot love and worship the Infinite. The intellect must be developed along spiritual lines; the will-force must have vanquished the animal cravings which are ever exerting a pull downwards. "The torch of wisdom must be lighted in the secret chamber of your heart." The soul must contemplate the glories of the Infinite Intelligence. Then, the love-force,—"the all-consuming fire?—shall inundate your heart. It will make your whole being vibrate in tune with the Infinite.

The student of Yoga is taught to meditate upon the Supreme Ruler of the Universe: Omkara! Why? Because to meditate thus is the highest worship. But that I have no power to teach. What is worship? There is the worship of Ignorance—Avidya; again there is a worship of the intelligence and illumined soul—the true Philosopher—the Gnani—the worshipper of the Om!

The worship of the worldly man has back of it the all-consuming forces PECUNIOMANIA.

Is then worldly happiness the proper standard to judge religion by? You may roll in riches. You may dine off the most succulent viands and the most richly prepared dishes. You may wear the costliest raiments. You may drive in the smartest equipages. You may live in palatial buildings adorned with the most beautiful appointments. You may have all the physical comforts such as the rich mines of Golconda or the artifices of modern civilization could procure you. The world may call you blessed by the Lord and you may lose your mental poise under the subtle influence of their fulsome flattery and indulge in heroics, may even consider yourself God's beloved. But stop. You are a pleasure-seeker; and the pleasure-seeker is an ass and so are they that pander to his vanity. If you think sense-gratification the *summum bonum* of existence, please stop reading this—it is not meant for you.

I just now mentioned a peculiar word—Pecuniomania. Now what is the significance of this word? Why, my friend, it is a disease. It is very infectious. It is a force that plays off man against man. Why does one fly at the throat of another? Why should be this blinding clash of human wills? Why should one man be so phlegmatic, so indifferent to the actual needs of another? Why should there be a constant feeling of hungry stomach, a parched throat and a feverish brain? Why should you so persistently talk evil behind the scenes of the very man whom you just now flattered face to face? Why should you consider the whole world selfish and feel yourself bound to blacken your soul through selfishness and deception? Take your mirror in hand and now just study your face. You are already on the hunt for that which will help you to gratify these cravings that the face portrays and that something is money. You are already a worshipper of the Golden Calf. You are praying to Plutus—the god of gold. This is pecuniomania. This thirst for gold to gratify the demands of your animal soul is a madness that dulls the eyes, stupefies the senses, coarsens the features and dwarfs the intellects of the young and the middle-aged as well as the old; women as well as men. Well may such as these feel utterly taken aback when there comes among them a man who, although young, opens his lips only to utter words of wisdom; opens his eyes only to look the living embodiment of perfect chastity and good will; seems utterly innocent of self-seeking, self-glorification, self-righteousness and self-importance. Did you ever see a man whose earnest enthusiasm and noble aims, shine in his eyes, dwell in the ring of his voice, seem to have entered his hands and feet and compel his entire being? These are true devotees of the Supreme Intelligence.

Such alone can pray. Prayer is the sincere lifting of the soul to the source of All-power. Prayer is the burning desire of the soul to achieve inner wisdom. Prayer is the earnest strain upwards of the intelligence to pierce the dark penetralia of Ignorance. Prayer is the ceaseless pressure upon the Superconscious mind—the Divine part of ourselves—to expand our sphere of insight. Prayer is the deepening of the intellect and the expansion of the Heart. Prayer is the triumphant conjunction of Reason with Intuition. Prayer is the cry of the purified and expanded soul for power and Wisdom to help and uplift, to purify and ennoble, to exalt and strengthen those towards whom it may feel itself drawn by the bond of spiritual affinity. Prayer is the longing of the son to co-operate with his father; to lift on his own shoulders a little of the heavy Karma of this world. Prayer is the struggle of the soul to free its wings; the flutter of the heart through the awe of lofty Idealism; the instinctive leaning on our secret selves; the drawing inwards for more light and life. Prayer is the concentration of the spirit on the Problems of the Divine life; the turning of the search-light of the Super-conscious-self upon the riddles of existence. Prayer is the filling of inner vision with positive light—light that rends asunder the veils of Darkness and Maya. Prayer is the souler-ascent up the magnetic chain of Evolution. Prayer is the meditation on the Infinite in the silence. Prayer is the faith of the seer in his visions; in his contemplation of the facts of life, inner and outer, subjective and objective, from the highest standpoint, in the utmost trust that he reposes in the Infinite; law that sweetly and steadfastly seeks to ever provide our feet with iron shoes for rough roads. "Prayer that craves a particular commodity—anything less than all good—is vicious. Prayer is the contemplation of the facts of life from the highest point of view. It is a soliloquy of a beholding and jubilant soul. It is the spirit of God pronouncing His works good. But prayer as a means to effect a private end is meanness and theft. It supposes dualism and not unity in Nature and in consciousness. As soon as the man is at one with the God he will not beg. He will then see prayer in all action. The thoughts of the purified soul are all prayer. Perhaps you will ask: What are the effects of prayer?

The attitude of the praying mind is one of intense concentration. The feelings which are the motive power of all men, have been wrought up to a state of tension. The nerve-currents are all being carried up to the brain and there converted into thought-power. With each exertion, whether mental or emotional, there is an outgoing current of magnetism. There sets up a stress in the ether. The entire organism is subject to Self-Magnetization. The psychic atmosphere around the praying soul is throbbing with his thought-forces. The aura—the photosphere round each form is bathed in living light, sending forth waves of golden yellow color and scintillating with unimaginable splendor. The finer forces of the super-physical planes have been attracted to you. Your mind is opened to the influx of Divine Help. Receive it. It is yours for the asking. The question of how to pray need not trouble us much. Prof. James, in his well-known work on "Psychology," makes the following most truthful remarks: We hear in these days of scientific enlightenment, about the efficacy of prayer and many reasons are given us why we should not pray, while others are given us why we should. But in all this very little is said of the reason why we do pray, which is simply that we cannot help praying. It seems probable that in spite of all that science may do to the contrary, men will continue to pray to the end of time, unless their mental nature changes in a manner which nothing we know should lead us to expect."

Quite so. It is your nature to pray. You eat twice and there are some who eat every three hours in the day, lest your body should starve. But in the meantime you are starving your soul. The moment you feel the need for a higher plane of Development, you will pray. Plato advised those who prayed to remain silent in the presence of the divine ones, till they remove the cloud from the eyes and enabled them to see by the light which issued from themselves." Apollonius always isolated himself from men during the "conversation" he held with God and whenever he felt the necessity for divine contemplation and prayer, he wrapped himself head and all in the drapery of his white woolen mantle. (Isis Unveiled P. I.) "When thou prayest, enter into thy closet and when thou hast shut thy door, pray to thy Father in secret," says the Nazarene. Prof. Hiram Erastus Butler—one of the noblest amongst the modern American Christian thinkers—says in his beautiful book, "The Seven Creative Principles:" "When heavenly desire is active, then man prays, but not without it can he pray effectually. Then the prayer of that soul which looks out upon the human family and the world and sees the fallen condition we are in today reaches out with that pure thought which they should have. O, for Wisdom and Power, that I might work under thy guidance for the elevation of my brethren; of those under my care! O, that I might become an instrument in the hands of that Infinite Power to work that I may alleviate, elevate and strengthen; that I may bring my fellows into the consciousness of that glorified life."

Now, reader: understand, once for ever, prayer is willing. It leads to the accomplishment of your aims on the spot. The righteous and pure soul expresses its will force in prayer. Thereby it is exalted into the spiritual realm. In this sphere Will is the basal power of influence. It draws all your finer forces into a focus towards the thing willed for. The result is that the thing is done. The astonished and grateful recipient attributes his success to a Special Providence and he is justified in doing so. The Great Law operates always and everywhere. The prayer simply attunes himself thereto by taking intelligent advantage of nature's forces. By prayer you come into rapport with the spiritually conscious side of yourself. You are as a needle pointing to the magnet—the more faith—and faith comes from Knowledge and Chastity—you put into the task, the sooner will you adjust your forces; the quicker shall be the response; the more lasting and powerful the reaction. Here, then, you have all the switches and levers of energy and inspiration.

Therefore pray ever and believe that your prayer shall ripen to fruition. Build up faith in the unseen and the invisible. The self in you is your guide, philosopher and friend. It is the Rock of the Ages—the Eternal among the Transient—the Source of All-Power, Wisdom and Activity. Lean on it for it is Strength—Invincible Strength.

THOUGHT: CREATIVE AND EXHAUSTIVE

THE right exercise of thought-power is an act of creation. "Each thought is a soul," says Lytton. "What you think that you are, what you shall think that you shall be," are the words of Buddha. "We live in that state of development our thoughts create for us." "A drop of ink makes millions think"—and one might pile one saying above another to the same effect.

The action of thought manifests itself continually. The power of suggestion and auto-suggestion, reigns supreme here, there and everywhere. Nations are caught up by an idea and their destiny is shaped thereby. A thought becomes the ruling passion of a man's life, and monomania or perfection in a certain direction is the natural sequence. One man meets another, and the latter's inner consciousness rises in response to the idea held in the former's mind and vice versa. No words have yet passed between them and yet the thought of each is known to the other. "Hide your thoughts?" says Emerson, "you may as well try to hide the suns and the stars."

Every one, who watches his thoughts, realizes that ideas as they enter our minds are accompanied by corresponding forces in their train. As soon as a thought comes in, there is an inrush of force in correspondence with it. This may be due to the calling up of other mental images lying dormant within the deeps of our mind, but which wake up as soon as they recognize an associate and hasten to combine with it. Different waves are thus stirred up in the mind. A peaceful thought is akin to the fragrant breeze of fresh air; a hateful thought is loaded with corroding influences. Let us illustrate the point:

My soul is filled with love or compassion for some one, man or beast, and my whole heart goes out thereto. I quite forget myself. A poor, stricken beggar, with tottering limbs and feeble form, catches my eye. Instantly a train of thought is started. I feel for him and with him. Pity and sympathy make me feel for him. Introspection makes me feel with him. I transfer my soul into his and feel the acuteness of his feelings. I live his life for the moment. And what is the good of having so lived his life? This—I have expanded. Something of the grosser side of my nature has been shaken out of me. Again some one has perhaps outstripped me in my mad hunt after money, or crossed me in a love affair. My whole being is a-quiver with rage and mortification. There is fire in my veins. "O, if I could catch the rascal on the hip! Ye gods, how I hate the fellow." I stamp my feet, gnash my teeth, and clench my fists. I am angry. I hate. Oh—Yes, decidedly. I know it. I have lived. But to what end? This—I have contracted, I have passed through two distinct moods, the one was creative, the other exhaustive. Which shall I choose?

All life is a flux of moods. The mind of man is continually vibrating. External impacts impinge upon it and galvanize it into activity. Impulses initiated from within act upon it. This ceaseless activity of the mind, if controlled and toned up to an exalted level, will at last lead us to that by knowing which man knows everything; if left alone, will knock us about here and there, from pillar to post, till, weakened and exhausted, we fall within the iron grips of King Death to be taught perhaps harder lessons hereafter.

The mind is like a wild, unbroken colt and requires to be broken in. So long as the waves of this mind are not stilled, the path to peace may not be trodden.

The law of action and reaction holds good everywhere. Between man and man, between brain and body, between the physical and supra-physical, between atom and atom, a constant interaction of energies is in full swing. Nothing goes out from us but must complete the circuit of its influence and come back to us. From within, outwards and then back again—that is the law of "Shristi:" projection.

We cannot stir up different conditions in the world of thought or of action, and yet escape free from the influences thereof. We cannot commit violence without having the causes which motived the act react upon us. Take an India rubber ball and throw it with force against a wall. The ball returns to your hand with exactly the same force which drove it through space to the wall. This is very simple.

The human brain may fitly be compared to a galvanic battery, generating currents of electric force, weak or strong, according to the nature of its structure and power. We generate a thought-current, bring it up to a high pitch of vibration, project it over our nerves and then off at the extremities, into physical manifestation; an act, a word, or something else. That is how I understand it.

The brain, which is a concentration of fine nerve matter, commanding an area of upwards of 300 square inches, when stimulated by a thought, generates force in the brain-cells, which number about 50,000 to the square inch; and currents of this force run down the nerves, which in turn are attached to these cells—the "brain" battery cells, we may well call them. Indeed physiology teaches us that attached to each cell are nerves, never less than two in number and sometimes as many as four. Minute nerve fibres proceed in bundles and cords from the microscopical centres, the cells—I mean,—all over the physique. These fibres are very fine, I may say, superfine, in structure, since their ultimate ends are not perceptible even under the lenses of a microscope. You may imagine how fine they are when I tell you that the smallest part of them, the microscopically visible part, "is calculated to measure in size not more than 1-15,000 part of an inch," and it is considered by advanced physiologists that even these minute nerves may after all be bundles of fine nerves. Now you may well conceive of the effects produced by an intense emotion, a powerful suggestion from outside, or a strong thought vibrated upon from within, upon the nerves which concentrate themselves mostly in the intricacies of the nervous system and generally all over the system.

The nervo-vital force, the psychoplasm, as some have wisely termed it, is in a state of exchange between the brain and the body. Each thought is of atomic origin, otherwise its transmission through the ether would be quite impossible. Each atom draws upon another atom for momentum, and therefore the energy of thought-atoms is vibrant in its nature. The finer the atoms which go to compose a thought, the more tremendous the rapidity with which they are whirled into action from within outside, and reaction from outside within. The nobler and more intense the thought, the greater its vibrant fineness and the wider its field of activity.

A calm ascension of the mind is perfectly compatible with a strong, sensitive, and glandular organization capable of standing immense strain, and registering on its sensitive nerve-wires the feelings and thoughts of those who come into contact with it. It can exercise the projective functions of the mind with a serene power. It can re-polarize the minds of weak, worried, suffering mortals by its mere presence. It can receive beams of spiritual light that flash downwards into it in the form of intuition, genius, and inspirational messages from the unseen. Remember, please, all this means everything and nothing for us just as we watch and control each mental tremor and quiver caused within us by our thoughts or drift along aimlessly cycle after cycle of our existence.

The human body is a channel for the influx and efflux of various forces and the degree of its purification shall determine whether much shall manifest in it or little. We live in the state of development achieved by the mind and the body—not muscular development necessarily. The body which is built up of the gross constituents of animal flesh and alcohol is hardly fit for employment in lofty thought and the spiritual evocator—he who calls the sacred spirits of the finer planes—sits stark naked and specially purifies his body that nothing impure should cling to him within or outside, lest he should, by the coarsened nature of his body or garment attract maleficent beings to himself. The mind cannot be tampered with without injury to the body and vice versa. Remember your entire physical organ is a thought-form, coarse or fine according to the quality of your thoughts.

Certain thoughts exhaust the life-force, others create it. Injurious thought-currents can be suppressed by raising an opposition wave. Hatred should be replaced by love, worry by hopefulness, hesitation by decision, anger by calmness and so forth: the finer always suppresses the grosser, mark you.

Training is necessary. Knowledge must be gained. Strength of the will-power must be developed. Now for a glance at the practical side of the question. For we have to acquire knowledge and then patiently see to the practical application of it in life. Mere intellectual contemplation of an idea is not the proper way to success in Occultism.

The mind is capable of existing in two states—Positive and Negative. Both are necessary for the up-keep of mental and physical equipoise. We must be able to call up either state at will and without the least of friction and strenuous effort. The positive state is a state of tension, alertness, centrality. The negative state is an attitude of receptivity, relaxation and non-resistance. The former if sustained all through the day would mean exhaustion and nervous breakdown. The latter, unless self-induced, would render us a victim to the "world, the flesh, and the devil." The former calls for an increase of nerve-force. The latter conserves this force and replenishes the store house.

We must attune ourselves to both these states. Thought is the fine cause of action; control the one and you have controlled the other. Evil, health-destroying and will-weakening thoughts must be faced by a calm and positive attitude. A position of strength should be taken up. "I am strong. I am pure. I have nought to do with evil thoughts and practices. I command my brain. My body is my slave. I am master within my own house. No thought here remains without my permission. No thought grips me and holds me its slave. I am master." By a calm positive attitude I mean that you should not allow yourself to be flurried and disturbed when faced by an Evil thought, but should face it as if already sure of conquest.

Simultaneously with these auto-suggestions, the attention should be turned to something lofty and noble. We must go on encouraging the inflow of noble ideas, till, at last, the evil thought is cut off from our mental vision and drops off altogether. The mind can think of one thing at a time. Think nobly and loftily and the evil thoughts will soon "take the hint" and cease to disturb you.

Whilst we repeat mental suggestions, we must feel their action. We must take long, caressing breaths and breathe life upon them. Thus they will become permanent in our constitution. With each successful effort, automatism will be hastened, till at last in a very short time we shall become so strongly grounded in our principles that bad thoughts will be thrown off automatically and nothing evil shall touch us. Express the Good the Pure, the Powerful in yourself and you can easily repress the Evil, the Impure and the Weak.

How easy to be good and pure, after all. Yet we spend years in fighting an evil and exhausting thought, when healthy mental occupation would throw its own blissful mantle of peace upon us. It is the only lesson I have learnt:—"Would you have peace? Then spiritualise yourself," and I give it to you with all the love in my heart. The more spiritually developed we are, the stronger and hence calmer we shall be. There is no doubt of this.

The Negative mental attitude is absorbent of energy only when it is given free play deliberately.

When seated at the feet of one, pure-hearted and loving; when studying the inspiring words of some great teacher; when under the influence of calm thought; after a strong and continued exercise of willpower, we ought to "relax," and receive the transmissions of energy from such sources, and breathe them in with a prayerful heart.

When praying to the Supreme Creator, let us be receptive of the currents of spiritual force that follow in the wake of devout prayer. The sun shines upon the dung-hill as well as the beautiful rose. The saint as well as the sinner can open themselves out for an inflow of divine energy by simple, earnest prayer. He who says otherwise is born blind. Science must repair the evil science has done by recognizing the efficacy of prayer. The negative state must be accompanied by an interior balance of mind.

The most important factor in the training and development of mind, in the expansion or rather the enfoldment of the soul, is Concentration.

Now concentration means the power of holding the mind to centre;—to a focal point, without allowing any other thoughts to touch you. Concentration is perfect attention. All, Yes! all possess this power of attention. We all pay attention to what we like. But the secret of strength lies in concentrating our minds upon what we do not care for. Mr. Raghavachary says in his beautiful little book, "The Magnetic Aura"—"Mental energy when forced into difficult and lofty channels develops Power, when allowed to run along lines of least resistance breeds weakness." I am quoting from memory, but that is the idea—the will must learn to concentrate upon what Mr. Raghavachary says if followed, would develop your mental muscles and will-power, wonderfully. All my readers should study this little book.

The element of "attraction" predominates. Let us utilize it. Suppose there is a hard bit of work a man does not like but which would be of great use to him if properly accomplished. What ought he to do? He ought to dwell on the advantages that would accrue to him if he did it. Thus at last what was dry work would become interesting, because he now knows it will make him happy. He should at first lead on the mind by gentle suggestions, then transmute the mood to a Direct Action of the will, remaining immovable and resolute.

Control of speech, control of action, control of thoughts—that is Self-Control par excellence. Resolve to succeed in this and every morning renew your resolve and act up to it. At first you will have some failures; but never mind; go on and you will succeed according to the strength of your Resolve.

We ought to decide upon the particular type of thoughts that should find an open door in the precincts of our minds. This particular set of thoughts must be encouraged, must be assimilated i.e., made part and parcel of our being, must be brought to bear upon our action and speech. "If you would be thoughtful speak thoughtfully," says an esteemed friend, Prof. H. E. Butler.

Each act must have a well-defined basis and should be seen complete mentally previous to being externalized. Forethought must precede action. Decision and tenacity of purpose should accompany its performance. A complete decision of the mind clears the mental field and is really the battle half won, at times, wholly won.

Each utterance must be well-grounded on a clear thought. It should be based on a strong conviction if it is to tell. Calmness and not muscular exertion of the larynx should accompany speech.

Silver-tongued men are always sweet tongued. Control speech, my friend. It is a mighty power. Let it not wound.

Each evil thought once entertained with delight sets up a magnetic centre for the attraction of similar others. It must be excluded promptly and a good thought substituted in its place. This must be done with tireless zeal till our mind will automatically repel the evil and welcome the good. For the law of automatism reigns supreme in entire life. Serious, thought-compelling books should be studied and their teachings applied with resolution in our daily lives, if we are to be in magnetic trim with them. We should keep ourselves healthily occupied mentally and physically. We should keep ourselves well-in-hand emotionally; for emotions are a great force, but must be controlled before they can be utilized; otherwise they will lead to our destruction.

What, O Friend, is blind passion that you should be in its thrall? What is death that you should be afraid of it? Neither body nor mind, neither wife nor children, neither wealth nor worldly enjoyment;—nothing will make you happy. That is what we all seek! Happiness. And that is rooted deep within ourselves minus world, riches and all such other toys.

Escape from the illusion of forms, of senses, and of selfishness. Know "Thou are God—*ta twam asi*, O Swetaketu," and be free. Know that you are for perfection, Eternal Love and Service Free. Thus; increase your Spiritual Stature and realize God who alone exists. All is His. All is He. He is Truth, Existence and Bliss. Then let us worship Him by right action, thought and speech. The path is open to all. Every one is welcome to tread it. The sooner we do so the better for us as well as the world.

MEDITATION EXERCISE

1. I will be what I will to be. I "can" and I "will" be Free.

2. Locked up in my soul is All-Power,—All-Wisdom,—All-Love. My first, last and only mission in life is to give Explicit Expression to the Soul-Force—the All-Go(o)d—implicit in my being. I live for Self-Perfection.

3. I yield to no external agencies . . . be they human or non-human. He that fights for me is Within me and he is strength itself. My inner nature is a battery of irresistible force.

4. By the way of nothing I resolve to realize the Parambramhan—the Supreme Self—the Absolute, who alone exists away beyond Time and Space; beyond Cause and Effect, beyond Light and Darkness; beyond all relative manifestation.

5. I renounce all thirst for Life on Earth or in Heaven. I resolve to be cold to Pleasure and to be calm to Pain. I am "Desire-Free."

6. Henceforth I obey no Law, man-made or God-made, but what is sanctioned by my own highest Intuition and Inner Judgment. I am a Disembodied Spirit working, living and breathing for all that is related to me by Spiritual Affinity. I care little for this world with its thousand-cloven tongues of gratis advice, praise and censure. I can but obey my polarity. I want nothing. I seek Strength in Chastity. I seek Wisdom in the Silence of my own heart, which is assuredly the Seat of Divinity and the Fountain of all Virtue and Goodness.

7. I dedicate myself—body, soul and spirit to the service of the "Great Orphan"—humanity. I worship God by serving Man.

8. I resolve in this life, so to train myself, that I shall be a tremendous centre of Spiritual Force. My entire personality must reflect Divine Splendour. It must be a living and powerful lever to Uplift, Ennoble and

Purify all such as come into contact with me. I am a Spiritual Exemplar of greatness.

9. I strive for the Christ-Life, the Buddha-Life, and the Great-Lives whose touch has brought me Light of Knowledge.

10. I resolve to be serious, devoted and constant in my principles every moment of my life, awake or asleep; at work or at rest; in society or in solitude; in joy or in grief; in praise or in blame; in earth-life or. hereafter. I am determined that nought shall shake my purpose, which is unalterably fixed. By the sword of Knowledge I will cut asunder and dispel all fear, within and without.

11. I resolve to be Fearless. I deny the Power of anything, within or outside of my physical form, to . weaken me. I am resolved that my nerves shall be steady and obey my mandates.

12. I resolve to be Pure and perfectly Chaste, Clean, Contented, and studious. I shall by force of my Will-Power crush and starve out all sensual and unclean thoughts; and conquer, most thoroughly, "the lust of the flesh, the lust of the eyes, the pride of life." I am the embodiment of Continence.

13. I resolve to live above the animal stage, above the merely human stage, above all, as far as possible, that pertains to either or both. I resolve to live the Divine Life—which is not only superhuman but is above it.

14. I resolve to master my mind and body. The education of the Will and the Expansion of my spiritual Stature is the aim of my existence, since what appear to be trials beyond the endurance of common humanity can have no terrors for the Expanded Intellect of the Yogi. The dawn of Spiritual Greatness heralds the death of Pain. Pain fructifies in the soil of Ignorance.

15. I resolve to thoroughly master all the principles of Spiritual Unfoldment and to spare no pains for the acquirement of right Knowledge; since the emotion that is a constant impulsion to noble living and lofty aspirations is baffled in its efforts and becomes a source of Pain unendurable, when the Clear Light of the Intellect does not shine upon the Path.

16. I resolve to mount guard over Speech, Thought and Action, lest by recklessness or inadvertency I should, in any way, however slightly, sully myself Spiritually and thus give myself cause for self-condemnation. I resolve to put Emotion under the yoke of Reason.

17. I resolve to be Gentle, Quiet and Loving to others. My bearing towards others shall be one of perfect sweetness. I radiate the Supreme Power—the Love-Force—the Expansion of which shall be my constant endeavour and a source of all-bliss to mankind.

18. I resolve to be a staunch upholder of the Great Law of Compassion and Non-injury. From me there can be no danger to anything or anybody. I wish everyone perfect Soul-Bliss.

19. I resolve to hold myself ever Calm and Serene. I can never be a slave to worry, anger or any other emotional disturbance, I am Master everywhere and always, over everything and all conditions.

20. I am independent of the body and use same as an instrument. I am and have Eternal Life. I am a Soul indestructible and have a body. I am one with All. I am the All.

The following extracts are from the *Kalpaka*—published by the Latent Light Culture.

SILENCE—What is Silence? Silence is to keep quiet. It is a great thing to keep silent. It can be called one of the greatest accomplishments that man can attain. It is not only for the development of the soul or any unfoldment of the self that it is useful, but it is also beneficial for both work and rest. When you keep silent the brain works much more accurately and the action of the heart is more steady; a physical rest ensues as all the members of the body are quiet, relaxed and in a state of receptivity.

A man who can relax his muscles will get more rest in an hour than one who cannot relax gets in one full day.

When one is silent, a beautiful stillness prevails, and it is then you come into consciousness more entirely. What is it? It is nothing but the understanding of your relation with God. How to make this practical?

When you read this you feel an upliftment; you realize yourself to a greater extent; you have a truer consciousness of infinite things. Every step of this advancing realization induces stronger consciousness of. Power. What more practical proof than this do you want?

There is no limit to Truth. There is no limit to your Power. There is nothing impossible for you in this universe. You must first realize this fact. If you wish to attain Power, you must be full of desire and attention.

What is desire and attention? It is nothing but concentration, pure and simple. It is only when you open the avenues of your soul to the influence of the Spirit that you can have liberty—liberty from bondage. In short, know yourself.

OBSTACLES—I am the master of my own life. I can overcome all obstacles and gain dominion over myself and my surroundings.

It is my duty to count my blessings and brighten the lives of others around me.

I shall not sadden others by complaining and faultfinding.

Do you realize that comfort cannot be found outside of yourself? You do; and yet the whole world is sinning, suffering and sighing for it. Then why don't you enjoy it?

You wish you could, but you find you have so many things to do, and you barely find time to devote to yourself. You must understand there is no permanence except in Spirit. You must utterly abandon your old ways of thinking and of doing. You must set aside an hour every day for sitting in the 'Silence.' The intense forces of life operate in perfect silence. You must take that hour by force until it becomes a habit with you. You will have peace and control. Life will be worth living.

You are but a part of the whole. The whole is Spirit. There is only one Spirit, and God is Spirit. Therefore you are spiritual.

No kind of material trouble can affect the spiritual. Everything is spirit. Lo! you are a being having everything in you. What you want is within your grasp. You can be what you wish to be. All that appears to be obstacles to your advancement is false, and does not exist. Assert your Self and become the master of all.

REFLECTION—One of the most important elements that constitute success is reflection. It is more or less an exercise—intellectual exercise; by this the mind is cleared and the thought receives a greater impulse. "Read and reflect" is an adage worth remembering. Just take a piece of poetry; read it slowly; think of its various meanings; value the thought that could have suggested the piece; weigh each word in it and see what a clearness and precision is before you.

Now take your life; aye, a day of your life; say from morn to eve. Just when you retire for the night, recount each word act and deed of yours from morning till then. Think over each of them in an impartial light; see what a host of light—true light—is thrown, and everything in its right sense is revealed to you. If your recounting portrays your acts of the day in a light which would make you blush, turn over a new leaf and improve yourself.

Try this for a week and say whether you have become master of your actions or not. A rigid training along this line will make you pure and enable you to control yourself and this leads to success.

BREATH—The Bible says:—"And the Lord God breathed into the nostrils the breath of life and man became a living Soul."

Man cannot live without air even for a few minutes, whereas he can go without food and water for days together. Breath is the life of man. The whole mystery of life is centered in this Breath.

Every day we hear about proper ventilation and the great value of pure air. All this is good and right. Proper ventilation is highly desirable. Pure air is essential. Above all, the way of breathing is nearly as important as the quality of air you breathe.

God has created air in abundant quantity; it is the only thing pervading space. It sustains all lives by oxygen, its life-giving property.

The act of breathing not only helps you to draw oxygen from the air but it also helps to throw out certain poisonous matter formed in the body by the breaking down of the tissues. The blood has a duty to perform. It makes a complete circuit in three minutes; carries oxygen to the tissues for their upkeep and takes the poison from thence and throws it out through the lungs. This taking of oxygen and throwing out of poison is performed through breath. So here you see that slow breathing will take in more of the life giving oxygen and at the same time throw out more of the poisonous matter formed within. It is estimated that one-third of the poison formed in the body is thus thrown out of the lungs and the remainder through the bowels, skin and kidneys.

Has it ever occurred to you, dear reader, that breath plays an important act in your everyday life? Just try this when a crisis is forced upon you or when petty cares of life seem to assume abnormal proportions, by sitting quietly and breathing deeply for at least three minutes. You will see what a comfort flows to you and what a balanced head you have to solve all this.

All the greatest statesmen, the greatest generals, the greatest orators and the greatest thinkers have been the deepest breathers. Deep breathing promotes vitality and greatness. Ambition and aspiration both materially and spiritually are fulfilled only by breathing—breathing in the proper way.

It has been accepted that there is something else in the air than oxygen—a life-giving, vitalizing property which the chemists have not been able to detect or analyse. It is Prana. You see that plants around you, aye, the whole vegetable and mineral kingdoms draw their life out of this air and live upon it. You know that vegetables and minerals have life. What is this life? It is nothing but Prana. Science has proved that men can subsist on air without food and water. Many experimenters have tried this, and most of them have been able to fast 40 days together with no kind of food and drink except air—pure air. They have not lost their weight. We have now in India many Yogis who live mainly on air not for days and years but for ages together. Why? Because they know how to breathe and draw sufficient Prana from the air to keep up the physical body.

What is Prana? Prana is Spirit. It is alive and conscious. The air or atmosphere is full of this vitalizing, living, conscious Spirit substance—the breath of life, the source of all life and energy.

Concentrate on this Prana, when you breathe the breath of life. You will see that your subconscious mind opens to receive this Prana. The mighty secret of the miraculous power of Yogis lies in the conscious reception of PRANA. Hence learn to breathe.

SELF-DE-HYPNOTISATION

IN the foregoing papers, I have tried to enforce upon my readers the indispensable necessity of shifting our point of view from the lower to the higher planes of thought-life.

It may be with regard to our physical self or our intellectual self or our emotional self;—we must view and manipulate them all from but one standpoint—the plane of the Spirit. This is one of the most important principles of Yoga. Yoga means Union. The human will trying to come into the plane of the Divine Creative Principles practises Yoga. The Creative thought in the Divine Spirit must of necessity exist in our minds. Then why do we not act up to it? Why are not our efforts directed purely to the working out of the great plan? Why, if we are really Divine, do we grovel in the puppet-play of a false worldly life?

The answer is we have been thinking invertedly. We have been basing our conclusions upon the suggestions of the sense-born intellect—the mind of the Flesh. We have to pass from this standpoint to that of the Spirit—God—the Absolute. We have to translate our highest conception of our relation to the Spirit into conscious values. The mere grasping of this relation would tend to their objective manifestation in us, through us and for us. A great saint of India said "the Summum bonum of Bodily existence is to realise in the human body the Supreme Personality of God;" that realisation is the magnum Opus of human existence and it is possible only when we transcend the Lower self and develop a correct appreciation of the spirit of the Great Will.

Man never creates anything; but when he seems to do so what he has done is this: He has specialised the Universal Energies under the directive power of his illumined intelligence by giving certain suggestions to the Universal Creative mind, which takes up the suggestions and moulds out the form from the Universal substance. Thus knowingly or unknowingly we are ever sending forth suggestions into the Creative Mind which at last start up before our vision as objective realities. From this we conclude that the Perfect thinker alone can create Perfect Forms; others must of necessity fail in this task. Hence our object is to come into conscious touch with the Perfect thought which gave the initial movement that developed this Universe. To accomplish this means the reproduction of the Perfect thought in ourselves. For the Universal tries to find expression on the plane of the Particular. Indeed this is the motive behind evolution, the development of individualised centres of consciousness resting in perfect recognition of their relation to the Absolute. Each soul is the centre of consciousness; a ray of Divine Light shot into matter; a reflection of the Divine Mind. These centres of consciousness must develop the Cosmic consciousness.

What is Cosmic Consciousness? It is the actualization of the relation which the part bears to the whole. The reader must not commit the blunder of supposing God to be capable of being parcelled out into parts. So we are not thinking of material things along lines of physical observation, but of that which is behind matter—I mean spirit—which is the Life that ensouls material forms and of which those fauns are simply so many projections. Suppose we place two mirrors facing each other—a large one and a small one. Suppose further that the word "Life" is engraved on the former; then by the law of reflection the same word shall appear in the latter. That illustrates the relation between the human and the Divine minds. Another illustration given by a mental scientist is that of a self-influencing dynamo where the magnetism generates a current which intensifies the magnetism thus leading to the generation of a still stronger current till at last the saturation point is reached. Only between the human and the Divine minds there is no such thing as saturation point, but the recognition of the latter by the former simply renders the former a medium for the specialization of the latter. Now suppose any illustration of the two mirrors, a quantity of dust accumulates upon the small one. Then, necessarily, no reproduction of the image on the large mirror can take place, in the small one. By evident analogy if the human mind is clouded it cannot awaken unto a realization of the Divine thought-image existing in the mind of the perfect thinker—God.

That is exactly our trouble. We are labouring under the hypnotic spell of thoughts not in consonance with the true spiritual laws of the Universe as well as our true self. This is the result of the inversion of thought. We have been under the impression that from external conditions we can develop inner stage of consciousness. This is the master-spell which is an illusion or Maya. Our entire thought-life has been rusting under the vitiating, poisoning effect of this idea. This is the poison seed which has developed the mighty tree of Maya. To pluck it out we must draw inwards and realise that inner states of consciousness wield an evermoulding influence upon matter and hew out ever varying forms, just as the image projected upon the specular screen of a magic lantern is really determined by the slide in the lantern. Change the slide images and you have other images on the screen. Change the thought in your mind and you change the form materialised thereby. Influence the lower self from this standpoint and your thought-life shall take on newer, more beautiful forms—which in reality form the grand and noble stuff composing the life of every highly evolved soul. The self has de-hypnotised itself from the illusion of forms. It has found its place in life—sees itself as the principle of life and is free and immortal.

SELF-DE-HYPNOTISATION—II.

The way is long; yet despair not, awake, arise and stop not until the goal is reached—Katha Upanishads.

LIFE is a constant accumulation of Knowledge. The vast majority of humanity are the pushed and a few are the pushers. The latter class have learned to grip the good in everything and turn it to account. Some have lived to purpose in the world of matter, some in that of Spirit. They do not seek, but are sought after, do not weep but are wept for; do not want but are wanted. They have gripped this Lesson:—Knowledge is power and Power moves the world. They have acquired knowledge by inner concentration upon certain problems and then applied the same with a cautious, a straight aim, and they have hit the mark.

Such indeed is the result of the right exercise of Knowledge. Now knowledge has many aspects. Some strive for the material side. of things, some for the Spiritual; ninety-nine per cent of the former to one of the latter. No blame is attached to either class. We must all of us follow our own bent. We are for the Spiritual and will therefore see how we can live the Positive Life from the Spirit's viewpoint. We are like so many pearls strung upon a band of gold. The band of gold is the great Universal spirit and each pearl is a point, a centre of consciousness in and through which the Spirit is trying to realize Itself.

We are half devil, half divine. Sheathed in our coat of flesh, our powers hooped in by the physical form, we cannot expect to come face to face with the Infinite. But there is within us, behind us, before, above and around us, God's Spirit, and we can realize our relation to it by putting ourselves En rapport therewith. To accomplish this grand event "to which the whole creation moves" the East Indian practises Yoga, and so gradually unfolds his spiritual consciousness.

We have tried elsewhere to give our readers a faint idea of this subject. Let me give you a few lines from a leading writer. The great distinguishing character of this stage is his consciousness of the Oneness of All. He sees and feels that all the world is alive and full of intelligence in varying degrees of manifestation. He feels himself a part of that Great Life. He feels his identity with all of Life. He is in touch with all of nature. In all forms of life he sees something of himself and recognizes that each particular form has its correspondence in something within himself. This does not mean that he is bloodthirsty like the tiger, vain like the peacock, venomous like the serpent. But, still, he feels that all the attributes of these animals are within himself—mastered and governed by his Higher Self—but still there. And consequently he can feel for these animals or for those of his race in which the animal characteristics are still in evidence. He pities them but does not hate his brother however much that brother's traits may seem undesirable and hurtful to him. And as he feels within himself all the attributes of the higher Life as well as the lower, he realizes that he is unfolding and growing into these higher forms, and that some day he will be like them. He feels the great throbbing life of which he is a part to be his life. The sense of separateness is slipping from him. He feels the security that comes from this consciousness of his identity with the All Life, and consequently he cannot Fear. He faces today and tomorrow without fear, and marches forward towards the Divine Adventure with joy in his heart. He feels at home, for is not the Universe akin to him—is he not among his own?

Such a consciousness divests him of Fear, Hate, condemnation. It teaches him to be kind. It makes him realise the Fatherhood of God and the Brotherhood of Man. It substitutes a "knowing" for a "blind belief." It makes man over and starts him on a new stage of his journey, a changed being.

No wonder that one in this stage is misunderstood by merely intellectually advanced people. No wonder that they often consider him to be a man functioning on the plane of Instinctivity, because he fails to see "Evil" in what seems so to them. No wonder, that they marvel at his seeing "Good" in things that do not appear so to them. He is like a stranger in a strange land and must not complain if he be misjudged and misunderstood.

But there are more and more of these people every year—they are coming in great numbers and when they reach a sufficient number, this old earth will undergo a peaceful revolution. In that day man no longer will be content to enjoy luxury while his brother starves,—he will not be able to oppress and exploit his own kind—he will not be able to endure much that today is passed over without thought or feeling by the majority of people.

And why will he not be able to do these things? may be asked by some. Simply because the man who has experienced this new consciousness has broken down the old feeling of separateness, and his brother's pain is felt by him—his brother's joys are experienced by him—he is in touch with others.

From whence comes this uneasiness that causes men to erect hospitals and other charitable institutions—from whence comes this feeling of discomfort at the sight of suffering? From the Spiritual mind that is causing the feeling of nearness to all of life to awaken in the mind of men, and thus renders it more and more painful for them to see and be aware of the pain of others because they begin to feel it, and it renders them uncomfortable and they make at least some effort to relieve it.

The world is growing kinder by reason of this dawning consciousness, although it is still in a barbarous state as compared to its future condition.

The race today confronts great changes—the thousand straws floating through the air show from which direction the wind is coming, and whither it is blowing. The breeze is just beginning to be felt—soon it will grow stronger, and then the gale will come which will sweep before it much that man destined for the ages. And after the storm man will build better things—things that will endure.

Have you noticed the signs—have you not felt the breeze? But mark you this—the final change will come not from Hate, Revenge or other unworthy motives—it will come as the result of great and growing Love—a feeling that will convince men that they are akin; that the hurt of one is the hurt of all, that the joy of one is the joy of all—that all are One; thus will come the dawn of the Golden Age. (Ramacharaka's Advance Course in Yogi Philosophy).

This then—the Spiritual Consciousness and the enfoldment thereof—is the motive prompting to the practice of Yoga. Some start in for practice before they have realized this aim. They have seen, heard of, read of some one possessed of Psychic Powers and their morbid tendency to sensationalism has fired their imagination. They are anxious to possess these Powers and rule their brother-man. They are anxious to make others tremble before them. They are anxious to strike terror to the hearts of others. These men do not know that they are taking a blind leap into the dark and terrible chasm of Black Magic. They do not know that any thought or action which consciously or unconsciously intensifies the sense of separation; causes friction between man and man; causes pain to the souls of others and lights the Hate-Flame of anger and impotent fear in their brains, is a retarding force and exerts a tremendous pull downwards upon their evolution. Such a motive has in it the germs of selfishness and the dark powers of black passion. Such a motive will bring untold pain, suffering and ignominy. It is the result of a Rajasic nature, where the intellectual powers are strong and the glow of passions arising from the desire to rule is fierce and destructive. These are the followers of the Left-hand Path. Their wills are strong as iron, their natures intense and implacable, their hearts cruel and devoid of gentle feeling, their passions seething and persistent. Yet all these will and must be shattered to tiny bits when set against the Great Will which is first the Fount of Love and Compassion and then bids everything to be governed by the Law of Love.

The modern craze after hypnotism has a dark side to it. Back of all hypnotic influence there is the subtle power of suggestion, personal magnetism, a powerful personality; and all these things are purely and simply the results of organized thought-Force and a trained Will-power. Now these two forces, namely thought-force and will-power, govern all the universe. When they are spiritualized, that is to say, when their action is subjected to the controlling influence of the Law of Love, they command an irresistible position. They strike where daggers fail,—of course, they may as a rule work both ways, for good or for evil, and, in either case, their subtle power makes itself felt. However, this subject is very wide and not within our province. I simply want to call attention to the pitfalls of Hypnotic Power and warn you against making use of or allowing yourself to be controlled by any such malign and insidious influence.

Now you who read this might view it all from a sensational standpoint and wish to practice hypnotism, although, of course, I do not believe it, for if you desire such power, your character must be dwarfed and Yoga is a path bristling with thorns for a selfish man. But student, sternly curb and kill out by determined and scientific training all such propensities. They are daggers to stab you, thorns to pierce your feet; they are the efforts used by the order of Black Magicians to retard your evolution. Before entering this Path, weigh, measure, gauge and study your character and build it up along spiritual lines, and these false desires will vanish as the mist before the sun.

While commenting on this great sin—the sense of separateness—these words in the Light on the Path ring in my ears. Let me quote them in full: "Seek in the heart the source of evil and expunge it. It lives fruitfully in the heart of the devoted disciple, as well as in the heart of the man of desire. Only the strong can kill it out. The weak must wait for its growth, its fruition and its death. It is a plant that lives and increases throughout the ages. It flowers when the man has accumulated unto himself innumerable existences. He who will enter upon the path of power must tear this thing out of his heart. Then the heart will bleed and the whole life of the man seem to be utterly dissolved. This ordeal must be endured. It may come at the first step of the perilous ladder, which leads to the path of life; it may come at the last. But, O Disciple, remember that it has to be endured; and fasten the energies of your soul upon the task. Live neither in the present, nor in the future, but in the Eternal. This giant weed cannot flower there; this blot upon existence is wiped out by the very atmosphere of Eternal thought."

The first duty of the initiate is to guard against this "Source of evil"—which is really the sense of Self-righteousness and the exalting of our own personality above that of others. It is refined animalism. It is intellectual pride and Egoism. Its climax is Black Magic—the giant weed. It belongs to the lower part of ourselves—the passionate side of us, from which proceed hatred, jealousy, malice, desire for revenge, self-glorification—and these tend to the setting up of a dividing wall between man and man. We contract ourselves by such practices. We are thereby building up a shell around the soul, which it cannot transpierce. You who take so keen and deep an interest in the Occult forces of nature will, by the study and practice of Yoga, in time develop a higher form of consciousness, far above the average of humanity. Naturally this unfoldment will transmute your inner nature into a tower of strength and your mesmeric influence shall gradually circle out from a smaller to an ever larger sphere. This is inevitable. Then comes the crux of the situation. Will you develop a Will that is potent with the strength of the All-God? that is flexible at need; rigid at need; ever strong to save and motived by the highest, the best and the noblest within you? When that great spiritual giant, Sri Ramakrishna Paramahamsa was lying very ill at the Cossipur Garden, Pandit S. T. is reported to have said to him "Sir, I have read in the Shastras that Saints like you can cure diseases of the body at will. You will be free from all your ailment if only you concentrate your mind upon the Spot—Ramakrishna Swami was suffering from cancer in the throat—with the will that it be cured. Won't you try it once? Now listen to the noble reply of this perfect soul. "O, how could you say such a thing, being a Pandit yourself? Can I ever be inclined to remove the mind, that I have given up to Sachchidananda—the Essence of knowledge, Existence and Bliss—from Him, and turn it to this frail cage of flesh and bones?" This is renunciation.

It is a general law of Occultism that the White magician should never use his powers for the accomplishment of personal ends, thus striking in at the very root of selfishness. In India the Spiritual Healer will not even drink a glass of water from the hands of the man whom he has treated. "I want nothing for myself." This is his calm, dignified and cheering speech. In the presence of such a man the lion and the lamb shall play together. The most vicious of brutes shall roll in submission at their feet; the most wicked men shall be struck dumb with awe and reverence on contact with their pure and spiritual aura. Nought out of or in the universe can injure them. This is the great power that shields the Yogi in the densest jungles of India. He is a centre of Love and Power and he knows absolutely no fear. It is the thought-magnetism of such men that brings immediate and complete relief. They are strong as rock. They raise not their hand against anything and nothing can go against them. They are living examples of the Law of Non-injury. This mighty power of Love, compassion and Non-injury is deeply imbedded in our nature. Encourage it and it shall grow. It is our very nature. After man has run the gamut of all ephemeral and sensual experiences, he falls back upon this heaven of peace.

"Look for the flower to bloom in the silence that follows the storm, not till then. It shall grow, it will shoot up, it will make branches and leaves and form buds, while the storm continues while the battle lasts. But not till the whole personality of man is dissolved and melted—not until it is held by the divine fragment which has created it, as a mere subject for grave experiment and experience—not until the whole nature has yielded and become subject unto its higher self, can the bloom open. Then will come a calm such as comes in a tropical country after heavy rain when nature works so swiftly that one may see her action. Such a calmness will come to the harassed spirit. And, in the deep silence, the mysterious event will occur which will prove that the way has been found. Call it by what name you will. It is a voice which speaks where there is none to speak; it is a messenger that comes, a messenger without form and substance—or it is a flower of the soul that has opened. It cannot be described by any metaphor. But it can be felt for, looked after and desired even amid the raging of the storm. The silence may last a moment of time or it may last a thousand years. But it will end. Yet you will carry its strength with you. Again and again the battle must be fought and won. It is only for an interval that nature can be still."—Light on the Path.

The blooming of the flower is the silence in the Spiritual awakening we have already spoken of. We have to concentrate our attention upon this. The first step to this illumination is Love. This is Bhakti Yoga—the religion of Love. "Love God with all thy heart, with all thy soul, with all thy mind and with all thy strength." And "thou shalt love thy neighbour as thyself." This is Love. No maudlin sentiment; the intense, burning love of the heart which sees all as one. No man who is a slave to love's opposite—hatred—can have Mukti—Freedom.

Then there is Karma Yoga. He who has lost the self has gained the self. This is the Yoga of unselfish action; service to others, men and animals, for the mere joy of it. The worker cares not for results, cares not for himself, but goes on putting forth his energies for the sake of others. It is selfless, sustained action in the interests of humanity.

In Raja Yoga, the mind of man, concentrated inwards, becomes Self-illuminated. The Raja Yoga is the master of mind par excellence. He sifts the grounds of psychology, develops his mind, purifies, trains and controls his nerves, opens up the centres of force in his body, conveys same into the brain and finally transcends it. He then goes on conquering plane after plane of consciousness till at last there comes a stage when he feels as if he were Everything and everywhere. This is Illumination—Samadhi—and when the Yogi has achieved this he has achieved all. The eternal Pilgrim—Man—has trodden the vast cycles of existence and come back home. The son has been united to the Father.

Gnyana Yoga is the Yoga of Wisdom. Here the intellect is at its best. The philosopher, the logician, the man of Reason, have their work cut out for them here. They must split hairs of argument, gain knowledge of the workings of matter, Energy, Force, mind-substance, and reasoning the interaction of these, finally arrive at an intellectual conception of the Absolute.

Let me add here that the reports of the intellect are by no means to be condemned as inevitably fallible as some philosophers have said for when your intellect contemplates some special line of thought for some considerable length of time, there pours in from the intuitive side of your consciousness—the Larger consciousness as some psychologists have called it—a flood of light which reveals all facts connected with that field of thought.

Once a philosopher met a mystic and when after an interview they parted, the philosopher said "All that he sees, I know" and the mystic remarked "All that he knows I see." We must develop all round. Unless a man's intellect is illumined by Gnyana, he cannot have any conception of the Riddle of the Universe; unless he has this knowledge he cannot realize his relation to the absolute. He is as a man groping in the dark. He cannot, in the absence of such recognition, experience the joy that surely results from the love and service of humanity—for the Lord shining within, changes the face of this world; shows me how I am one with others and by no means different; until the Higher Self unfolds through the training of Raja Yoga and dominates "the lust of the flesh, the lust of the eye, the pride of life" no progress is possible and progress in the control of the Lower Self comes only through Raja Yoga.

It is time we came to the proper appreciation of this fact. Turn once again to the Light on the Path and read this attentively and follow it. "Seek it not by any one road. To each temperament, there is one road which seems the most desirable. But the way is not found by devotion alone, by religious contemplation alone, by ardent progress, by self-sacrificing labor, by studious observation of life. None alone can take the disciple more than one step onwards. All steps are necessary to make up the ladder. The vices of men become steps in the ladder, one by one, as they are surmounted. The virtues of men are steps—indeed, necessary—not by any means to be dispensed with. Yet though they create a fair atmosphere and a happy future, they are useless if they stand alone. The whole nature of man must be used wisely by the one who desires to enter the way. Each man is to himself absolutely the way, the truth and the life. But he is only so when he grasps his whole individuality firmly and by the force of his awakened spiritual will, recognises this individuality as not himself, but that thing which he has with pain created for his own use, and by means of which he purposes as his growth slowly develops his intelligence, to reach to the life beyond individuality. When he knows that for this his wonderful complex and separated life exists. Then indeed, and then only he is upon the way. Seek it by plunging into the glorious and mysterious depths of your own inmost being. Seek it by testing all experience by utilizing the senses, in order to understand the growth and meaning of individuality, and the beauty and obscurity of those other divine fragments which are struggling side by side with you and form the race to which you belong. Seek it by study of the laws of being, the laws of nature, the laws of the supernatural, and seek it by making the profound obeisance of the soul to the dim star that burn within. Steadily as you watch and worship its light will grow stronger. Then you may know you have found the beginning of the way. And, when you have found the end its light will suddenly become the Infinite Light."

Let the reader study and re-study this beautiful passage and formulate the ideals of his life along these lines.

The mental motive temperament, in my opinion, is the best fitted organically for the rapid unfoldment of spiritual susceptibilities. Here the lower organs of alimentiveness, Amativeness and Bibativeness are generally under the control of the Higher Brain Centres. Here the mind predominates over the body. Their emotions are vivid and intense. They possess great aptitude for mental activity such as is induced by no other temperament. Their physical constitution is equally fine and possesses an instinctive loathing for all gross and immoral practices such as bind a man's thought, to the physical and carnal side of life; their thoughts are quick, clear and lean to the idealistic side of things. They often overstrain themselves and are very impulsive. This class of men should live as much in sunshine and open air as they can. Their sex-nature also should be kept clean and pure from childhood. Parents should never hurt their feelings nor impose conventional doctrines upon them for they will never submit to any domineering and are generally considered "queer" by coarse-fibred people because of their meditative turn of mind. These are, if well-trained, or if simply saved form the society of immoral men, the best types of men. Their eyes are, as you may notice, almost always very expressive because they are given to abstract thinking and much idealism. If you belong to this class, do not think badly of yourself if the world does not understand you, for you are far advanced and have a much more highly-organized brain than men can in their present stage of unfoldment rightly appreciate. You must learn to control your emotions or you will find yourself tossed roughly about in this rough world. "You are" as a friend humorously put to me, "from another sphere" and your soul is seeking to view life from "finer" sense planes. Do not condemn yourself if people call you an impractical dreamer.

It simply means that the physical senses have little attraction for you and your introspective mood implies the stirring of finer sensibilities within you. Your indifference to worldliness is the result of satiety and I for one do not condemn myself on this score.

As knowledge of the inner life increases one finds but small reason for frequent self-condemnation. By this it is not implied that you should be proud and haughty and all that. Even such a thing as "spiritual pride"—the feeling of conscious chastity and psychic attainment—the "I am holier than thou" feeling—should be guarded against. Such a thing is sure to have its fall. Many so-called spiritual teachers who "spring up, grow, and then go to seed" are really victimised by this feeling. What is meant is that you should not hypnotize yourself into a false sense of undue humility, shyness and nervousness—things which sap your moral strength so that you cannot look another man in the face. Remember, friend, it is no sign of spirituality to allow others to dupe you, to "bite you in the face" and sit upon you. You should on such occasions stand up to such men and by your bearing give them to understand that you are by no means a vacuous fool or a brainless scapegoat, but that they must "keep off or you will wax dangerous."

Do not sit with or have anything to do with men who have no sympathy with your views. They must either come up to your level or they are welcome to go their way and leave you in peace. Do not go out of your way to correct others. Do not unnecessarily meddle with the affairs of people who are self-sufficient. Do not feel disturbed if people make fun of and scoff at your cherished ideals. Let them. It matters not. They do not realise the depth of their ignorance and hence their dogmatising, care-crazed peacock-like attitude. You may safely trust time to bring light to them.

Let me recall to your mind Hamlet's most truthful words. "Pure as ice, chaste as snow, thou shalt not escape calumny, and truly even the Great Christ was maltreated, so what of our puny selves."

The student should cultivate "Indifference." Many have complained to me of being forced by sheer pressure of circumstances to live in the constant society of men who are given to obscene and immoral practices.

I can quite understand the position of my friends. Such things are really painful to a growing soul and to avoid them thousands seek the forests of India lest "the world, the flesh and the devil" should awaken responsive vibrations within them and spoil matters. But all cannot do it and the time is fast approaching when the general race-consciousness shall take a higher range and obviate the necessity of such isolation.

However we may, for the nonce, call to our aid the habit of shutting ourselves up in absolute reserve when forced into such society. Do not let us hate them because that would be a serious breach of the Occult law of Love, but withdraw your attention and sit perfectly still. This is a good way of training your will-power and you should make use of it to the best possible advantage.

But should they by overt act try to shake you off your balance, then I do not see any harm in "putting up a fight" and when once driven to this step, do not desist till you have reduced your tormentors to final and unconditional surrender. All this may sound to some very "Unspiritual" but, "Even a worm shall turn," and I must warn my readers against the will-weakening habit of allowing others to make fools of them.

Hold your forces in reserve and turn them into proper channels. One of the society drills so common amongst men is to visit one's friends for a little "gossip" and an inane time of senseless laughter. Such a practice is declared to be a means of relaxation. But I solemnly warn and forbid my readers against all such forms of indulgence. Leave weak-minded fellows to think of such relaxation. You and I simply cannot afford to demoralise ourselves by such follies. However we hope to tell you a little more of all this in our next chapter on character building proper.

Men are like so many toys in a toy house. One blow and they go to pieces. It is not a bit of use covering a hideous carrion with a mass of roses. Our very love of God is often candidly speaking, the outcome of fear. As Judge Troward in his "Lectures on mental science" says: It is a hidden form of hate: and I endorse his statement. The eternal one has never given us cause to stand in awe of him. It is ignorance alone that leads from pitfall to pitfall, and Ignorance is the absence of Love. Let us then drill these facts into our brain. Let us think these thoughts till they become flesh of our flesh and the bone of our bone. Let us awaken the electrifying force of the Higher soul—the Atma—Shakti and Gnana—Drikshti—that alone can supply us with exhaustless force to wing the Spirit that would break its cage and fly to Peace which is Perfection.

Let O Student, the fire of the spirit course through your views. Nought can crush you. Drive and thrash out of your brain all thoughts of fear and worry. Know yourself and thereby know everything. Be yourself and thereby be everything. Conquer yourself and thereby conquer everything. Tremble not at the task. That which quakes and quivers is of the flesh and yours is the grand onward march from Passion to Peace. Difficulties are only as a spur to effort. It is not the greatness of a difficulty so much as the feebleness of our spirit that bars our progress. Face them and they fly. Quail not. Quail not. These things touch not the Permanent self. They are the incidents of our relative personality. There is never a rigid barrier between a difficulty and its breakdown. Square your shoulders and apply them to this wall of Illusion. See how it vanishes before you. I say again: Be yourself: Know yourself: conquer yourself: trust yourself: and nothing can long ensnare your manhood.

CHARACTER-BUILDING

KNOWLEDGE gives power. Power controls. Man stands for inner perfection. Our character is the sum-total of our inner unfoldment. What is unfoldment? I told you in my paper on Spiritual Unfoldment of the different bodies of Man and how the right control and culture of each body would enable the light of the Spirit to stream forth to the objective plane of existence in all its pure radiance. Here is a beautiful illustration. Take a small but strong, electric light bulb wrapped around which are many pieces of cloth. Suppose further that the electric light in the glass bulb is the Spirit shot into the Spiritual Consciousness in and through which the Spirit can shine out without the least obstruction and with a minimum of resistance. Remember the Light is the spirit and the glass bulb is the thin veil of brilliant mind—substance known as the spiritual mind. The piece of cloth immediately next to the glass bulb is very fine and the light pierces it through. The piece of cloth next to this one is a little less fine and receives a little less of the light. Thus each piece of cloth as you go lower and lower is less fine than the one immediately next above it till at last you come to the last piece. This cloth-piece is at once the thickest and the least illumined of all others. You will see that whatever bit of light this last one has is all it can possibly receive. Compared to this piece, the last but one is brighter and more desirable and so on from the bottom upwards. As you take off piece after piece, more and more light comes to you and when you have stripped off the entire number of cloth-pieces you have the pure electric light shining out of the transparent glass bulb. Need I tell you how the last piece of cloth is the physical organism. The grossest and least lighted-up sheath of man. The ego is mounting upwards as it were, from the densest veil of matter to more and more rarefied grades. The more rarefied the grade of matter in which you are clothed the more highly energized and spiritualized it is. The finer your body, the more powerfully vibrating the pranic force animating it. Think over it in connection with the illustration of the tiny, strong, electric light confined in the glass bulb and do not feel particularly attached to your physical form.

CHARACTER—CONTROL.

Let us in this paper confine ourselves to (a) Habit-control, (b) thought-control and (c) self-control.

I have already spoken to you, in full of thought-control in a preceding paper. I advise you strongly to master and apply the principles laid down in that lesson conjointly with what little I succeed in giving you here, for truly, Habit and thought are the two great pillars of our whole life-structure. They are the roots which sustain the tree of Life. Poison the roots and you have set your plans for the rapid corrosion of the royal tree; nourish and strengthen the roots and the tree shall grow, develop and expand; it shall put forth leaves, flowers, branches, and bear life-giving, sweet and nourishing fruits.

First of all let us consider Self-Control. What is it? How is this great virtue to be acquired?

What is self-control?

Self-control in Yogis is demonstrated by perfect Soul-Calm. A perfect Yogi will never allow himself to be cast into or hurried away by any form of emotional disturbance and excitement. Indeed the mere idea is absurd in connection with such developed souls. When they move through the restless and busy throngs of men yielding every moment to some emotional impulse; at times sad, at others glad, utterly unable to say a firm, "No" to their impulses; unable to view things from any higher point of view than that of the Relative and the transient form of existence and getting miserable and falling into dejection at the least touch of adverse conditions arising from the singularities of their unillumined intellects;—on such occasions the self-controlled man will remain unmoved in this atmosphere of conflicting thought-Magnetisms. While all sorts of thought-waves are dashing against him his mental aura remains untouched and unshaken, and he radiates peace. When he sees distress and pain, he does not make the whole air throb with his cries but he calmly sets about finding a remedy for the evil. When something goes against his personality, he does not give way to a blind rush of anger but he holds himself perfectly unruffled.

There was a great sage in India named Vyasa. His father, his grandfather and his great-grandfather had all of them struggled for Perfection and had fallen short of the mark.

Vyasa had himself striven for the same prize and failed. But as no honest seeking goes unrewarded, at last a son was born to Vyasa who was to manifest perfection in himself. Vyasa named him Suka. He taught him, trained him and initiated him into the inner mysteries of the Spirit. Suka was wonderfully intelligent. He soon grasped the principles of spirit and embodied them in himself.

In those days there was a great philosopher-king named Janaka. He was called "Videha"—bodiless, since he had lost all thought of body and believed himself to be the spirit. Vyasa sent his son to this king's court so that he might be put to test. Janaka being a developed occultist came to know of this intuitively and made suitable arrangements. When Suka arrived no notice was taken of him. The guards gave him a seat but otherwise were quite oblivious of his presence. This was no light matter. Vyasa was the most venerable sage in the country and could dictate to any one. But Suka was a Gnyani. For three days and nights he was left to himself. He sat there calm and serene.

Then they conducted him into a splendid suite of rooms. All sorts of luxuries, fragrant baths and regal honors were paid to him. Not a muscle of his face moved. He was calm, serene and thoughtful. This continued for eight days. Then he was led before the king who was sitting in full court. Music was playing. You know the intoxicating influence of music upon the brain. Beautiful girls and damsels, fit to bewitch the most abstemious of men, were dancing and singing. In short, it was a most impressive and splendid court. The king presented to Suka a cup of milk. It was full to the brim. "Go seven times round the court but spill not a drop of milk." Suka gravely bowed his head and accepted the cup. Round and round the court he went. Thousands of pairs of eyes were levelled at him. The music, dancing and nautch-girls of ravishing charm were all up in arms against his concentrated attitude of calm and repose. But this man went round, and after the seventh round returned the cup to the king—full to the brim—with the same quiet expression. The King, the court and everyone else could only gasp with surprise. This is the ideal self-controlled man. Naught could distract his attention. Can you conceive of a more positive proof of self-control? We shall do well to bear this story in mind and, whatever be our position in life, our gaze should ever be turned upwards and inwards. Never mind the form of occupation. Always maintain an inner balance and as soon as you are free, your attention should fly back with intense longing to the Higher Life.

WHAT IS HABIT-CONTROL?

Habit or automatism compels all organized life. Habit is a rhythm established by the Will. Now the former is Static. It works along sub-conscious lines of mentation. If you lift the brain-cap of man, you would see the belt of glowing and phosphorescent brain-substance physiologically known as the Corpus Callosum—this is the organic base of consciousness for the operation of mental energy. The finer the matter, the greater, the more powerful its vibrant force. This matter is constantly in motion, that is it ever vibrates.

Habit is a mode of motion. It is the same pitch of vibration repeating itself. The action of the Will is dynamic. When a man thinks concentratedly for some length of time upon some resolve, deep vortices are formed in the brain-substance. To these vortices the Will communicates a certain wave—motion which continues till the force which gave it the initial impulse exhausts itself. The stronger the will, the greater the wave-length and the more lasting its action and the deeper and more intensely active the vortices. You know how tenacious human nature is of habits. It cannot but be so. Your thoughts create these vortices. Your actions deepen them. Repeat the initiatory impulse and the Law of automatism will take it up permanently and keep up the motion. Your thoughts and actions register themselves in your brain-cells and nerve-force. Each inward tension of the Will develops changes in the molecular structure of the brain and since there is an immediate rapport between the brain and the nervous system that which exhausts or recuperates the "Volts" in that battery of vital powers—the organized human brain—welds a corresponding influence upon the vital centres of the body.

Professor Elmer Gates of Chevy Chase, the great American Experimenter in the new science of Psycho-Physics, who has been conducting experiments in an elaborate laboratory through complicated apparatus for measuring the sensations and emotions of man is of the opinion—and this opinion is endorsed by D. Carpenter in his grand work on Human Physiology and many other leading investigators on the subject—that every conscious mental activity creates in some part of the brain a definite chemical and anatomical structure; that mind-activity creates organic structure; that one essential condition of remembrance is the refunctioning of the structure which was originally created by the conscious experience which we remember; that organisms are mind-embodiments; that there is an art of brain-building and mind-embodiment whereby individuals can get more mind; that evil emotions create poisonous chemical products in the cells and juices of the body; that there is an art of promoting originative mentation, consciously and subconsciously; that immoral dispositions can be cured by putting in the same parts of the brain where they have evil-memory structures a far greater number of good structures, and then keeping the good structures functionally active a greater number of times daily than the evil ones; and that one's mental capacity can be more than doubled. The self-activity of the mind creates organic structures and, says Professor Gates:

"The mind rules the body. Here you have the grand principle of magnetic affinity between brain-waves and health-conditions in a nut shell. Psychologists give two divisions of the Habit-nature: the natural and the artificial. The natural is the mode of motion kept up by the Instinctive mind for the up-keep of health conditions. It is quite well-educated. Do not disturb it by trying to take control of it. The body has been abused and badgered by the artificial life of modern civilization. Go back to nature; have full confidence in it and do not meddle with the Involuntary activities of the body. As to artificial habits, I will simply say that they arise from the singularities of the ill-developed mind.

Remember this: All instinctive action is the continual and automatic swing of motion at first initiated by the Will and later on established on a permanent basis by continued repetition. This rhythm, if improperly and unwisely initiated can be swung on to a new line or can be disturbed. The will which started the motion can assuredly call it back by starting an opposite set of vibrations, which are finer and more powerful and bring about an equilibrium of forces and, by the further sustenance of same, develop an entirely new condition. One can change one's physical conditions as well as mental and emotional states by suggesting to one's subconscious mind the desired transformation and by constructing a mental picture, contemplating and projecting same into the realms of subconsciousness. As James Allen puts it:

Mind is the master-power that moulds and makes, and man is mind and ever more he takes.

>The tool of thought and, shaping what he wills,
>Brings forth a thousand joys, a thousand ills:

> He thinks in secret and it comes to pass;
> "Environment is but his looking-glass."
> We build our future, thought by thought,
> Or good or bad, and know it not
> Yet so the universe is wrought,
> Thought is another name for Fate
> Choose then thy destiny, and wait
> For Love brings Love, and Hate brings Hate—
> Again: All that we are is the result of thought.
> Lord Buddha: "The Dhammapada."

Now if you would control your habits, you must begin by forming Positive Decisions and then act them out. For instance, if you want to correct yourself of Fearfulness and Nervousness, sit quietly and repeat to yourself in all earnestness, "I resolve to drive out of my brain all fear thoughts. I will not permit them to come in. I am master. I am Brave. I am perfectly fearless. I resolve to be full of Courage, Snap, and mental vigor. I am Master."

Repeat this to yourself earnestly, concentratedly and positively. Insist upon immediate mastery. Say "I will conquer, this moment, this very moment," and set up the Strong Present tense. This is a most important fact to remember. When you sit down to concentrate, relax all over, breathe deeply and gently, and let your mind dwell exclusively upon these thoughts. Then gradually wind up your brain to a state of inner tension. Do not contract your brows. Do not clench your fists. Do not make any physical movement at all. Let the body rest in quiet repose. Let the mind be alertly poised. Set the teeth together quietly for the lock of the jaws is the seat of the will-force, but do not grind and gnash them. Simply close your eyes and shut out of your mental vision all the external world.

Retire into yourself mentally. Draw inwards. As the mind becomes tense, the body naturally follows suit. But this is not right. You should "break off" from time to time and then begin again. Soon the body shall be taught to lie quiescent while the brain is intensely active. Concentrate twice every day at the same hour. Soon the Law of Periodicity will set in and lead you into your room for your concentration exercise although you might have forgotten it. Be rigid in these matters. When you have once begun, do not be overcome by initial failures and your lapses into former states of mind. The new form of vibrations must adjust themselves along settled lines and you must persevere by right thoughts and their determined execution into actions till then.

Do not make false promises to yourself. If you do so you will become a miserable "dreamer" prostrated by mental weaknesses. Determine to do a thing and do it. After you have made your resolve to banish evil thoughts and crush a certain bad habit, turn your mind to Oppositely-higher types of thought and habit and persist in your resolve to be Master. Remember a resolve will last a certain length of time in proportion to the force which generated it and then it must be renewed repeatedly till it becomes clinched into a habit.

Hold firmly in your mind the particular thought which you would embody in yourself, during the time you are nourishing your body and at least an hour afterwards. This will liberate certain finer forces from the food and nourish particular brain-centres that you are building up. Do the same when walking in fresh air and when having physical exercise. This will deepen the thought-channels in the brain. Remember, at first there will be resistance from the lower brain-centres, but as the higher centres develop they will take absolute control. Go on. Stop not; you must build up a new brain in which the higher centres will control the lower ones and this process of Brain-transformation has to be done. It is very painful, but now that you know these things, and see the absolute necessity of setting about the task, it is no use getting impatient. The following lines from Dr. Sheldon Leavit, M. D., will help you immensely when practicing the above exercises. It has a direct bearing upon the setting up of the strong Present, I have already spoken of.

The present tense crystallizes possibilities. In "I am" and "It is" are wrapped great possibilities. There is a wealth of satisfaction to be found in being able to say, in all faith, "I am well, I am strong, I am Happy." Assurance like this crystallizes into tangibility, the things for which otherwise we are perpetually longing. It is a giant hand reaching out into the future and bringing to our feet what has long eluded us. Faith then proves a wonder-worker. It stands sponsor for us under all the trying conditions of life. When desire rises within us for some great good upon which to build a useful and happy life; the Present tense of faith at once brings it within our grasp.

To effect our purpose we should not hesitate to avail ourselves of the help to be had from any of the facilities at command. In a particular emergency all we lack may be the inspiration which shall drive us to triumph. Our greatest trouble arises from the tendency of the human (lower) mind to dwell upon failure rather than Success. We lose confidence in our ability to accomplish because we ourselves or some one else has met with failure, and it becomes necessary to churn up all our emotional energies to carry us past the sticking point. The best of us are not using a tittle of the powers which we really possess. Compared with what we ought to be, we are only half awake. It is right here that the power of assertion can do effective work in the rousing of our dormant faculties and bringing into strong action the forces awaiting our command. But they need vigorous stirring.

A young physician had been lying ill for many weeks from what appeared to be a serious complication of disorders, from which he had nearly given up hope of recovering. All his powers of resistance were seemingly in ruin. He could not sleep, he could not eat. He could not speak above a low tone. To sit up was beyond his power; his vital forces were at so low an ebb. His circulation was feeble and even his mind appeared to be wavering. After a careful examination I pressed upon him the need of summoning all his mental and physical powers, tottering to a final fall, in a grand effort to throw off the terrible incubus, which was crushing him as a strong man might crush his foe, by one vigorous and desperate effort. It did not seem hard for him to believe, under the stimulation that he would ultimately recover, but to bring his faith to immediate acceptance of relief was the difficulty. But he resolved to do this and warmly confessed his faith when at once the force of the ailment broke, the life-forces were set into cheerful and strong action and he soon resumed his place among men.

In reviewing the case I can see that it was that final culmination of all his hopes, that concentration of all his mental and spiritual powers into creative assertion, that lifted him out of the desperate condition into which he had sunk, and from which he would probably have moved downwards on gradually declining planes, to utter despair and death.

Before I close this chapter let me reiterate some important points. You can control your habits, however perverse they may appear. A complete decision of the mind is the first step. Effort, yea, Positive Effort and an indomitable will is the second thing. Remain unshaken in your resolves. Remember the first twenty-five years of every man constitute the Formative Period of life. The habits that you carry with yourself across this age become persistent and die hard. The psychological explanation is simple. During adult age growth is very rapid and your brain-channels are strongly grooved out; but this should not lead you to despair. You can render your brain responsive and pliant by earnest endeavor at any period of life, only those who take to these things in their youth will find the task of habit-culture comparatively easier. But it matters not at all whether you are young, middle-aged or old. You must do these things, not because of any extraneous pressure—you who have followed me so far cannot and should not believe in any such thing—but because it is the law of your nature.

At first when you start forming a new habit, there is resistance from your brain and many heroic efforts are necessary. Then gradually the task shall become easy and really pleasant. Another important fact to remember is that if at some hour today you go into your room and send forth an intense thought, next day the same thought shall start up in your mind at the same point of time. This is known as Periodicity. Therefore supposing you want to perform some difficult task with which your mind is not accustomed to cope, Sit up a few hours previous to that time and suggest to yourself, "I wish you, subjective mind, to prepare yourself for the performance of such and such a task tomorrow at 4 o'clock. Be sure you do it. Now prepare yourself." Next day you will find yourself quite prepared to accomplish the task. Suppose you wanted to get up at 4 o'clock in the morning. Before retiring to bed say to yourself on your subjective mind "Look here—I wish you to get up (or wake me up) at 4 o'clock. Be sure you do it." You will wake at that hour..

Always concentrate your attention upon such autosuggestions and repeat them till you feel sure your commands will be obeyed and they will be, if you insist upon their fulfilment positively and persistently with confidence. Believe in your power to succeed and everything in nature shall rush to your aid.

CONCLUSION

DEAR Student: Before we part let me thank you for having paid attention to what I have said thus far. This work is meant solely to extend to you a helping hand in the thickening gloom of Materialism which I see with horror and pain all around me. Whatever I have tried to tell you has received a trial at my own hands and may it strike a sympathetic chord in your heart. It may be my good fortune to present to you more fully some truths of the Grand Yoga Philosophy of ancient India of which I have hardly succeeded in touching even the outskirts. You may catch a passing glimpse here, a flash of light there:—but what of that? The Lord alone can enlighten your intellect. Therefore meditate and pray often and wait in patient earnestness for the dawn of spiritual Light from within. It will come. You cannot escape your own birth right.

Peace—Peace—Peace—be unto You.